Tibia

Relation of diaphyseal length and gestational week in the tibia

mm	Gestational week			mm	Gestational week		
	5%	50%	95%		5%	50%	95%
8	11	13	14	38	23	25	27
9	12	13	14	39	23	25	27
10	12	13	15	40	24	26	28
11	13	14	15	41	24	26	28
12	13	14	16	42	25	27	28
13	13	15	16	43	25	27	29
14	14	15	16	44	26	28	29
15	14	15	17	45	26	28	30
16	14	16	17	46	27	29	30
17	15	16	18	47	27	29	31
18	15	16	18	48	28	30	31
19	15	17	18	49	28	30	32
20	16	17	19	50	28	31	33
21	16	18	19	51	29	31	33
22	17	18	20	52	29	32	34
23	17	18	20	53	30	32	34
24	17	19	20	54	31	33	35
25	18	19	21	55	31	33	35
26	18	20	21	56	32	34	36
27	18	20	22	57	32	34	36
28	19	20	22	58	33	35	37
29	19	21	23	59	33	35	38
30	20	21	23	60	34	36	38
31	20	22	23	61	34	37	39
32	20	22	24	62	35	37	39
33	21	23	24	63	36	38	40
34	21	23	25	64	36	38	41
35	22	23	25	65	37	39	41
36	22	24	26	66	37	40	42
37	23	24	26	67	38	40	43

R. Schumacher   L. Seaver   J. Spranger

Fetal Radiology

A Diagnostic Atlas

Springer

Berlin
Heidelberg
New York
Hong Kong
London
Milan
Paris
Tokyo

Reinhard Schumacher
Laurie H. Seaver
Jürgen Spranger

Fetal Radiology

A Diagnostic Atlas

With 124 Figures in 202 Individual Illustrations
and 27 Tables

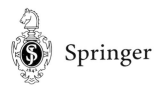

Springer

Professor Dr. med. Reinhard Schumacher
Kinderradiologie
Kinderklinik und Kinder-Poliklinik
Klinikum der Universität
Langenbeckstraße 1
55131 Mainz, Germany

Dr. Laurie H. Seaver
Greenwood Genetic Center
1 Gregor Mendel Circle
Greenwood, SC 29646, USA

Professor Dr. med. Jürgen Spranger
Universitätskinderklinik
Klinikum der Universität
Langenbeckstraße 1
55131 Mainz, Germany

Greenwood Genetic Center
1, Gregor Mendel Circle
Greenwood, SC 29646, USA

ISBN 3-540-20342-7 Springer-Verlag Berlin Heidelberg New York

Library of Congress Cataloging-in-Publication Data
A catalog record for this book is available from the library of congress. Bibliographic information published by Die Deutsche Bibliothek
Die Deutsche Bibliothek lists this publication in the Deutsche Nationalbibliografie; detailed
bibliographic data is available in the Internet at <http://dnb.ddb.de>

Springer-Verlag is a part of Springer Science+Business Media
springeronline.com

© Springer-Verlag Berlin Heidelberg 2004
Printed in Germany

Editor: Dr. U. Heilmann
Desk Editor: D. Mennecke-Bühler
Production: PRO EDIT GmbH, Heidelberg, Germany
Cover Design: Frido Steinen-Broo, eStudio Calamar, Spain
Typesetting: K. Detzner, Speyer, Germany
Printed on acid-free paper   21/3150Di   5 4 3 2 1 0

Acknowledgements

This book could not have been written without the help of many physicians who provided material for consultation. Our heartfelt thanks go to Horst Müntefering, who during his long tenure as head of the Department of Pediatric Pathology of the University of Mainz oversaw the diagnosis and classification of fetal material, securing the establishment of a remarkable collection of fetal specimens. We gratefully acknowledge the help of Dr. Tim Tralau, who faithfully assisted in the radiographic documentation and selection of cases. We are indebted to Springer-Verlag and ProEdit, notably to Dr. Heilmann, Mrs Mennecke-Bühler and Mrs Diemer, for their commitment, patience and expertise in producing this book.

Mainz/Greenwood   R. Schumacher
February 2004   L. Seaver
                                                                                    J. Spranger

Contents

Introduction

Intrinsic errors of skeletal development are individually rare but of clinical importance because of their overall frequency and their impact on patients' lives. Conventionally they are divided into *malformations* – defects of single bone – and *dysplasias* – systemic defects of chondro-osseous tissue. Depending on the type of surveillance system, limb reduction defects, one major category of skeletal malformations, are recognized in 3.1–6.9 of 10,000 newborns (Eurocat 2002; Makhoul et al. 2003; McGuirk et al. 2001; Stoll et al. 2000). Due to spontaneous or induced fetal loss, the prevalence in fetuses is higher, up to 15.7 of 10,000 (A. Queisser 2003, personal communication). The overall prevalence of neonatally manifested skeletal dysplasias is about 2 out of 10,000, half of them lethal (Andersen 1989; Cobben et al. 1990; Connor et al. 1985; Rasmussen et al. 1996).

As sonography has become a routine component of prenatal care, many of these disorders are diagnosed prenatally confronting family and physician with the question of elective termination of pregnancy. Ideally, this question is discussed on the basis of a specific diagnosis. However, such a diagnosis is difficult to achieve by fetal sonography. Even under optimal conditions it is missed in at least 35% of cases (Doray et al. 2000; Parilla 2003; Stoll et al. 2000) meaning that many abortions are performed on the basis of diagnostic suspicion.

Postnatally, the prenatal diagnosis has to be verified. To do this, fetal radiography becomes important. It is an effective, simple and economic way to establish a diagnosis or to narrow the number of diagnostic possibilities sufficiently to direct pathological, biochemical or molecular studies in their quest for a specific diagnosis. A specific diagnosis is required for various reasons. It permits sonographic quality control. It provides the clinical basis for research. More importantly, it is required for proper parental counseling. Parents who have gone through the termination of a pregnancy have a right to know all the available facts as to possibilities of recurrence.

This book has been written to assist in fetal postnatal radiological diagnosis. It is divided into three chapters:

1. *Development of the normal fetal* skeleton between gestational weeks 10 and 23. The chapter presents age-dependent standards with which to compare diagnostic films.

2. *Radiological differential diagnosis* of conspicuous defects of single bones such as pre- or postaxial limb deficiencies or vertebral segmentation defects. These malformations occur alone or combined in numerous conditions which are tabulated to assist in differential diagnosis. Starting from a given specific abnormality, malformation patterns can be recognized leading to a specific diagnosis or to a narrowing of the number of diagnostic possibilities.

3. *Fetal osteochondrodysplasias.* Skeletal diseases caused by factors that continue to express themselves after the earliest stages of fetal development result in osteochondrodysplasias, systemic alterations of form, structure, and maturation of bone. Recognition of the expression pattern allows for a specific diagnosis with its prognostic, genetic, and often molecular information. In this chapter are found illustrations of the salient radiological manifestations of the most common lethal and nonlethal osteochondrodysplasias manifesting in fetal life.

References

Andersen PE (1989) Prevalence of lethal osteochondrodysplasias in Denmark. Am J Med Genet 32:484–549

Cobben JM, Cornel MC, Dijkstra I, ten Kate LP (1990) Prevalence of lethal osteochondrodysplasias. Am J Med Genet 36:377–378

Connor JM, Connor RAC, Sweet EM, Gibson AAM, Patrick WJA, McNay MB, Redford DHA (1986) Lethal neonatal chondrodysplasias in the West of Scotland 1970–1983. Am J Med Genet 22:243–253

Doray B, Favre R, Viville B, Langer B, Dreyfus M, Stoll C (2000) Prenatal sonographic diagnosis of skeletal dysplasias. A report of 47 cases. Ann Génét 43:163–169

EUROCAT report 8 (2002) Surveillance of congenital anomalies in Europe. Ulster University

Makhoul IR, Goldstein I, Smokin T, Avrahami TS, Sujov P (2003) Congenital limb deficiencies in newborn infants: prevalence, characteristics and prenatal diagnosis. Prenat Diagn 23:198–200

McGuirk CK, Westgate MN, Holmes LB (2001) Limb deficiencies in newborn infants. Pediatrics 108:E64

Rasmussen SA, Bieber FR, Benacerraf BR, Lachman RS, Rimoin DL, Holmes LB (1996) Epidemiology of osteochondrodysplasias: changing trends due to advances in prenatal diagnosis. Am J Med Genet 61:49–58

Stoll C, Wiesel A, Queisser-Luft A, Froster U, Bianca S, Clementi M and EUROSCAN study group (2000) Evaluation of the prenatal diagnosis of limb reduction deficiencies. Prenat Diagn 20:811–818

Tretter AE, Saunders RC, Meyers CMK, Dungan JS, Grumbach K, Sun CCJ, Campbell AB, Wulfsberg EA (1998) Antenatal diagnosis of lethal skeletal dysplasias. Am J Med Genet 75:518–522

1 Development of the Normal Fetal Skeleton

Introduction

The fetal skeleton ossifies in a time-dependent sequence of patterns. The elements of these patterns – foci of mineralization within preformed mesenchymal templates – can be recognized by radiography and ultrasound.

Radiographic sequential patterns will be presented in this atlas using images of normal fetuses at specific gestational ages (Figs. 1.1–1.13). The images were selected from about 150 normal fetuses. Only those X-rays were used, where gestational age, clinical age based on foot length, and radiographic age were in accordance.

Recognition of a pattern of ossified structures allows the determination of the developmental stage of a given fetus within the range of normal variability (Tables 1.1–1.5). With few exceptions, variability ranges for the first appearance of marker bones, such as the ischial bone or the middle phalanx of the fifth finger, are not known. The standard error for the appearance of a specific ossification center is estimated to be approximately ± 1 week. Variability increases with gestation; it is smaller in a fetus of 12 weeks than in a fetus of 23 weeks gestational age. To add precision to this admittedly coarse estimate, age-related percentiles of the femoral length will be provided in the legends to the age-specific images. These are taken from published percentiles of normal femoral growth, which were obtained in population-based sonographic and radiographic studies (Merz 1988; Scherf 2001). In a normal fetus, pattern age (Eurin et al. 1993) and femoral length age will be identical. Lack of congruence points to developmental abnormalities. For instance, a femur length of less than 15 mm in a 16th gestational week fetus suggests intrauterine growth retardation. On the other hand, absent ossification of the cervical vertebral bodies in a fetus with a femur length of 22 mm suggests delayed ossification of the axial skeleton, as seen in some skeletal dysplasias.

The images of normally developed fetuses at specific ages will also provide the normative basis with which to compare abnormal looking bones. While crude abnormalities such as longitudinal or transverse limb defects, are easily recognized, discrete abnormalities such as developmental delay, minor formative and structural abnormalities of single bones or the entire skeleton, are not easily diagnosed without resource to abnormal features.

References

Eurin D, Narcy F, Le Merrer M, Maroteaux P (1993) Atlas radiographique du squelette fœtal normal. Flammarion, Paris

Merz EA (1988) Sonographische Überwachung der fetalen Knochenentwicklung im II. und III. Trimenon. Eine Studie über das Wachstum der langen Röhrenknochen im Vergleich zum Kopf- und Rumpfwachstum sowie über die Verwendungsmöglichkeiten der fetalen Knochenlänge im Rahmen der geburtshilflichen Ultraschalluntersuchung. Habilitationsschrift, Universitäts-Frauenklinik Mainz

Scherf W (2001) Normwerte fetaler Skelettmaße mittels post-mortem-Radiographie. Thesis, Humboldt-Universität, Berlin

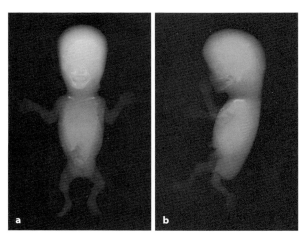

Fig. 1.1a, b. (Original size) *Week 9–10.* Length of femur: 2 mm
Milestone: The clavicles are ossified; there is no ossification of the vertebral bodies and the neural arches
Earliest ossification centers are seen in the clavicles, mandible and maxilla. The basiocciput, the orbital roofs and the ribs are faintly visible. Small condensations are present in the diaphyses of the long bones

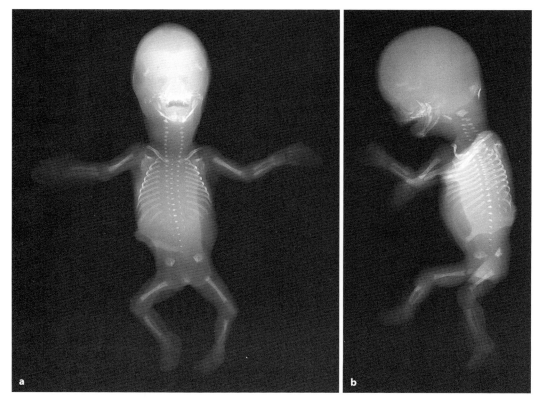

Fig. 1.2a, b. (Original size) *Week 11–12.* Length of femur: 7 mm
Milestones: The metacarpals and vertebral bodies of the thoracic spine become visible
Ossification centers appear in orbital roofs, the occiput, maxillae, and mandibulae. There is still a symphysis menti. The calvaria is not ossified. The clavicles grow toward their acromial ends. Ossification centers of the neural arches are visible from C1 to the upper lumbar vertebrae. The vertebral bodies are ossified in the thoracic and lumbar spine. Iliac bones and scapulae are seen as well-rounded structures. There is incipient modeling of the long tubular bones demarcating diaphyses from metaphyses. The metacarpals and metatarsals appear. The proximal phalanges of digits 2–5, both phalanges of the thumb, and one ossification center of the great toe appear

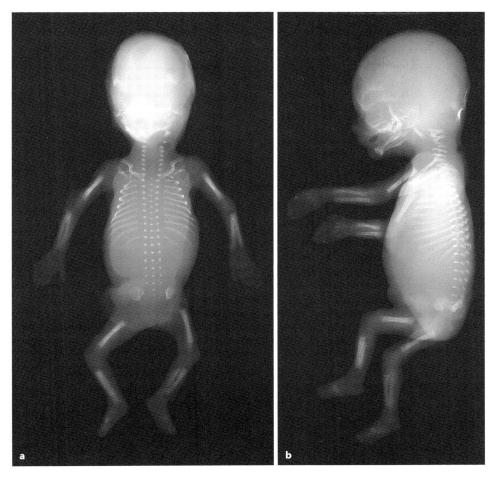

Fig. 1.3a, b. (Original size) *Week 13.* Length of femur 10–11 mm (normal range 10–15 mm)

Milestone: Ossification of the neural arches extends to the sacrum

Ossification of the zygomatic bone progresses and the lower lateral angle of the orbit becomes visible. The medial parts of the orbits are now delineated. In the lateral projection, a dot-like ossification dorsal to the orbits marks the lesser wing of the sphenoid bone. In the AP projection, they are faintly seen in the medial parts of the orbits. The clavicles have assumed their characteristic S shape. This fetus has 11 pairs of ribs. Neural arches have appeared in the lower lumbar spine and upper sacrum. The distal phalanges of the toes are visualized

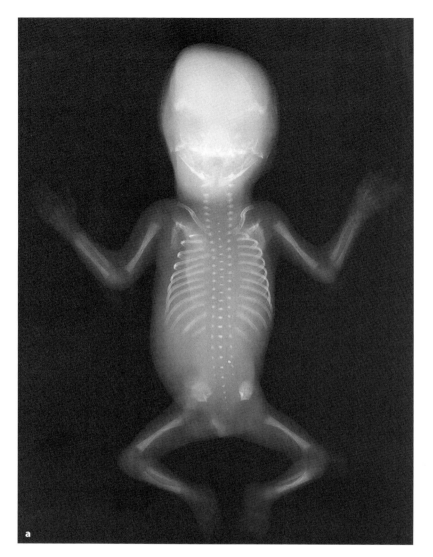

Fig. 1.4a, b. (Original size) *Week 14.* Length of femur 15 mm (normal range 10–18 mm)

Milestone: The nasal bone is ossified

The nasal bones are now ossified and the lesser wings of the sphenoid bone are more clearly seen. Sacral bodies 1–4 are ossified. The lumbar bodies have grown in their AP dimension. A coronal cleft or small notches in their upper and lower plates may be present. All phalanges of the fingers are ossified except the middle phalanx of digit V. In the feet the proximal and distal phalanges are inconsistently ossified

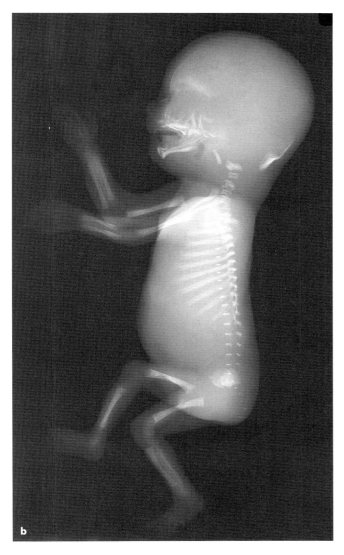

Fig. 1.4b

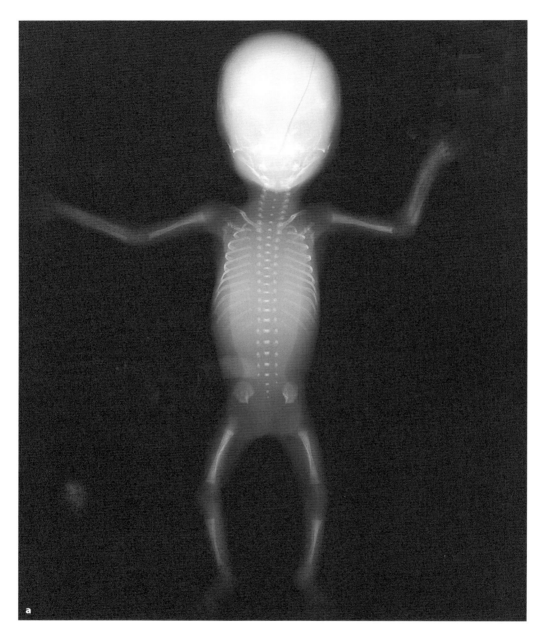

Fig. 1.5a, b. (Original size) *Week 15.* Length of femur 16 mm (normal range 12–21 mm)

Milestones: Ossification of the cervical vertebral bodies has occurred. Hand phalanges are more distinct

The maxillary palatine processes are ossified. The symphysis mentis is still visible. Ossification of the vertebral bodies is now complete from C3 to S5 with some variability in the mineralization of the upper cervical and lower sacral bodies. The coracoid process of the scapula appears. In this fetus all short tubular bones of the hands are visible – including the middle phalanx of the fifth finger. The proximal phalanges of the toes are more distinct

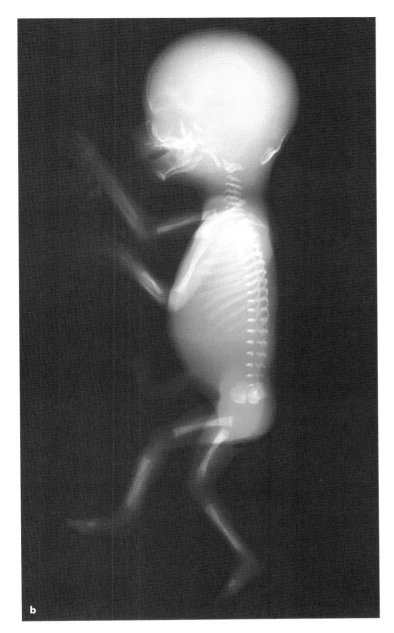

Fig. 1.5b

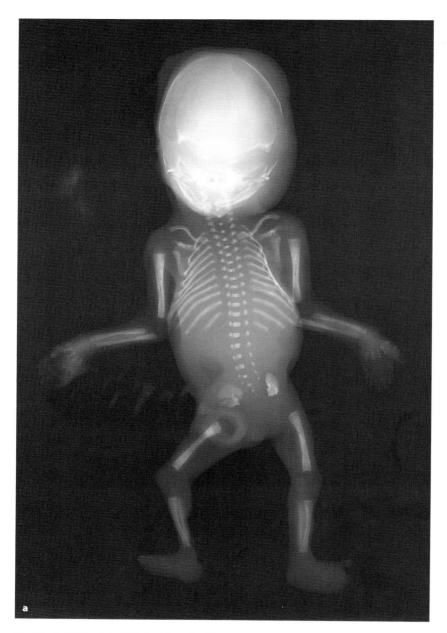

Fig. 1.6a, b. (Original size) *Week 16.* Length of femur 18 mm (normal range 15–24 mm)

Milestone: Ossification of the ischial bone occurs in 35% of fetuses

The lower nasal cavity is well modeled. In the anterior parts of the mandible and the maxilla the first tooth buds develop. A discrete angulation develops in the mandible. Both wings of the sphenoid are clearly seen. The vertebral bodies assume a more cubic shape and the AP diameter of the neural arches of the lumbar spine increases. The ischial bones become visible. The phalanges of the fingers are well visualized except the middle phalanx of the 5th finger. Ossification of the distal phalanges of the toes is variable

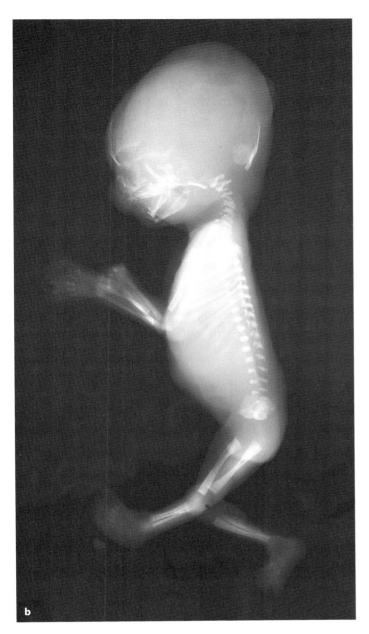

Fig. 1.6b

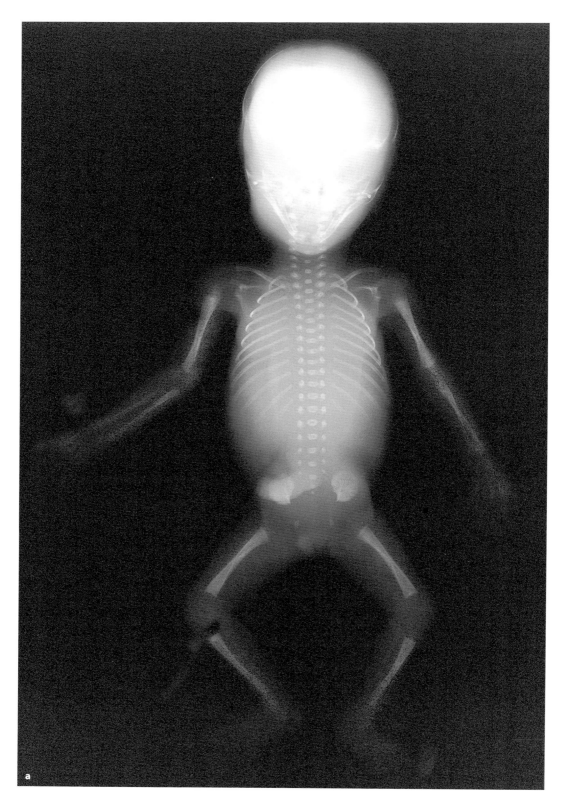

Fig. 1.7a, b. (Original size) *Week 17.* Length of femur 23 mm (normal range 18/27 mm)

Milestone: Os ischium is clearly visible (>95%)

In this fetus the vertebral bodies caudal of S2 are not yet ossified. In approximately 95% of fetuses the ischial bone is seen and assumes a more vertical orientation. The middle phalanx of the 5th digit becomes visible but is smaller than the distal phalanx. In the lateral projection the proximal metaphysis of the ulna is slightly angulated

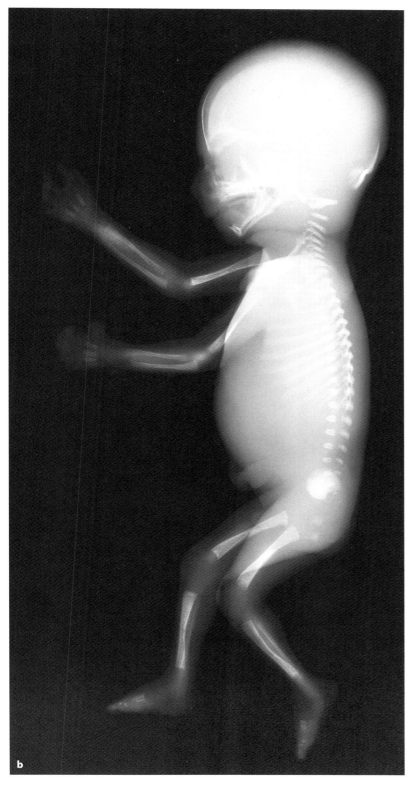

Fig. 1.7b

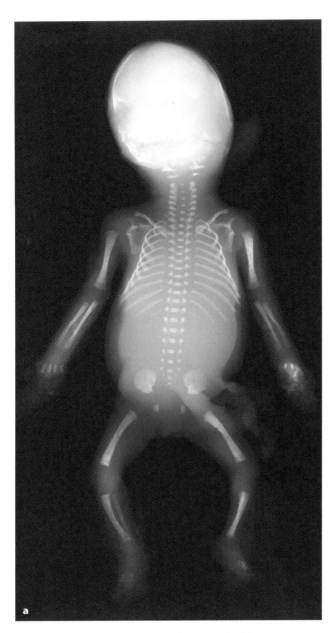

Fig. 1.8a, b. (75% of original size) *Week 18.* Length of femur 24 mm (normal range 20–30 mm)
Milestones: Body of S3 is always visible; angulation of the proximal end of the ulna is seen
The odontoid process is not yet visible. The body of C3, as well as the bodies and neural arches of S3 to S4 are now ossified. There is incipi-ent development of the lower ilium with a small osseous spur at the medial end pointing inward and downward. The proximal ulna is still slightly angulated. Cervical ribs and sagittal clefts of the upper tho-racic vertebral bodies are seen in this fetus

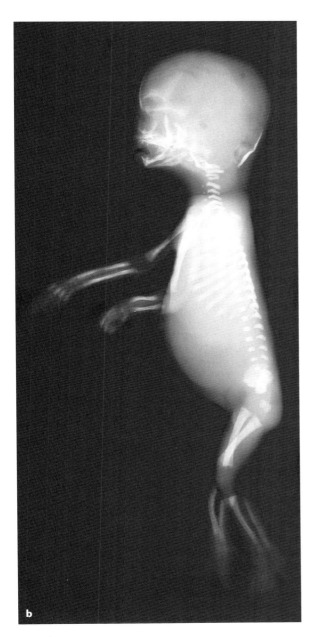

Fig. 1.8b

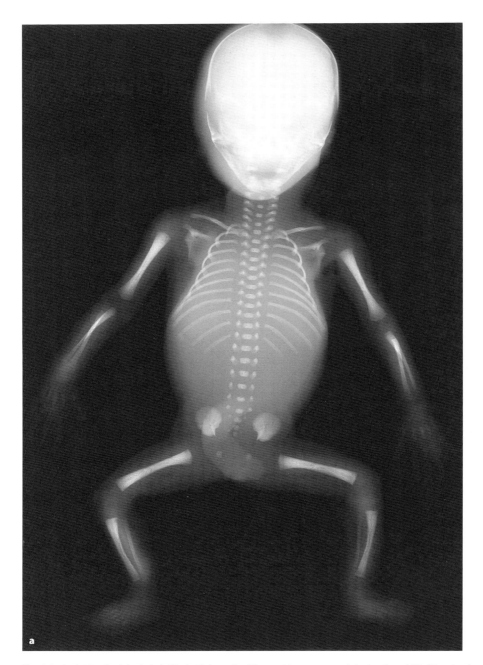

Fig. 1.9a, b. (75% of original size) *Week 19.* Length of femur 29 mm (normal range 23/33 mm)

Milestones: The tips of the upper incisors and the body of C2 become visible

The first tooth buds appear in both maxilla and mandible. Ossification of the cervical spine progresses with complete ossificati-

on of the bodies of C2-C7 and a decreasing distance between verte-bral bodies and arches. The odontoid is not yet ossified

Modeling of the proximal ulna begins to form a concave articular sur-face. The calcaneus is visible in about 13% of fetuses

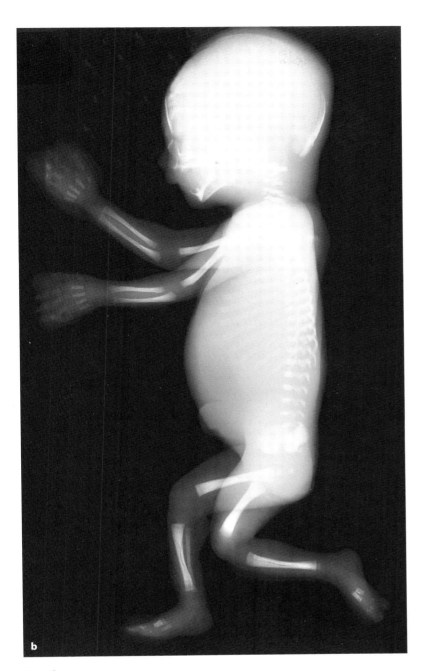

Fig. 1.9b

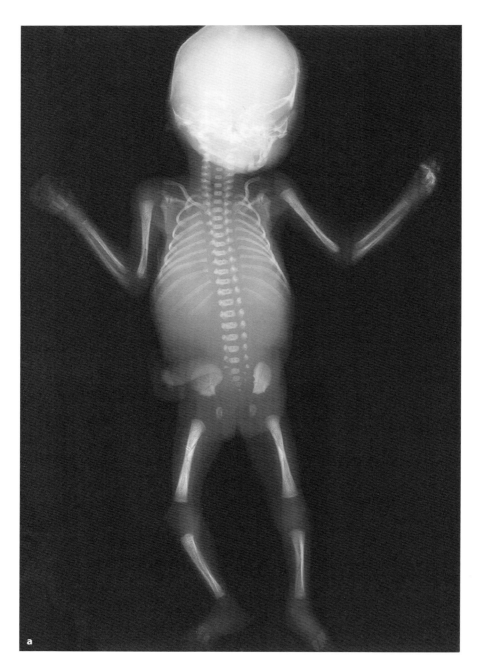

Fig. 1.10a, b. (75% of original size) *Week 20.* Length of femur 31 mm (normal range 26–36 mm)
Milestone: Tips of the incisors are regularly visible
The upper semicircular ducts are visible. Ossification of the vertebral bodies is complete from C2 to S4. A lateral indentation demarcates the iliac wings from the lower ilium. The acetabular roof is horizontal with a spur extending downward and inward from its medial aspect. The medial edge of the ischium is slightly concave. In the early maturing fetus the calcanei become visible. Modeling of the proximal ulna progresses to form a concave articular surface ventrally and a convex olecranon dorsally

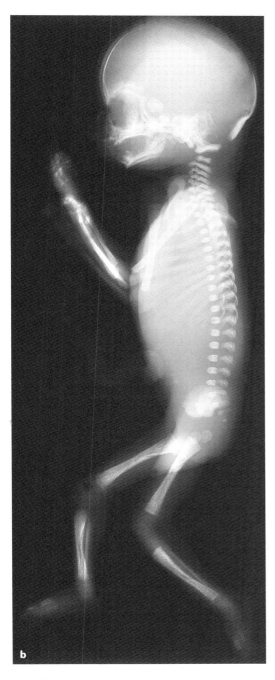

Fig. 1.10b

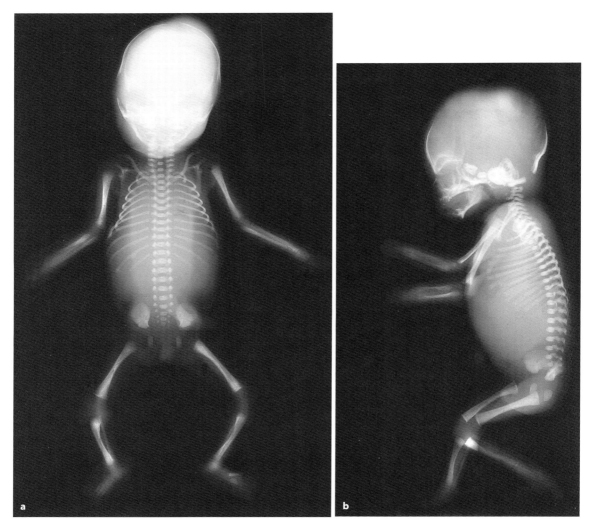

Fig. 1.11a, b. (Half original size) *Week 21.* Length of femur 36 mm (normal range 29–39 mm)
Milestone: There is an increased number of deciduous teeth

The vertebral bodies become more voluminous with a decreasing distance between bodies and neural arches. There is progressive thickening of the ischial bones

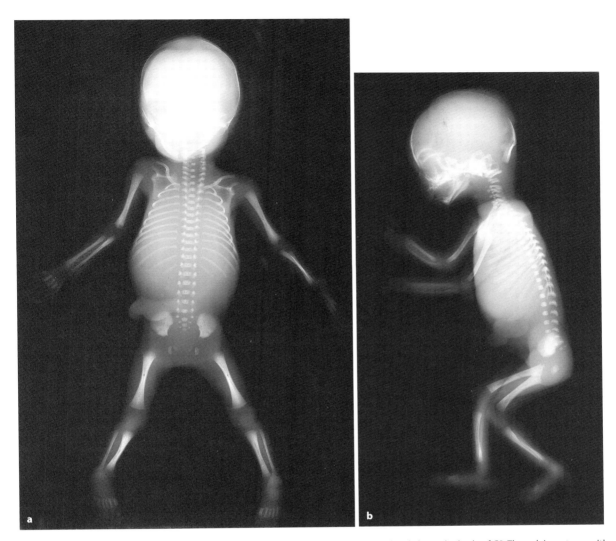

Fig. 1.12a, b. (Half original size) *Week 22.* Length of femur 35 mm (normal range 31–41 mm)

Milestones: Ossification of the odontoid process and pubic bone is seen More tips of the teeth are seen including the canines. The odontoid process is visualized above the body of C2. The pelvis matures with a distinct iliac body, disappearance of the downward projecting medial spur, and incipient ossification of the pubic bone. In this fetus, the calcaneus is not yet ossified

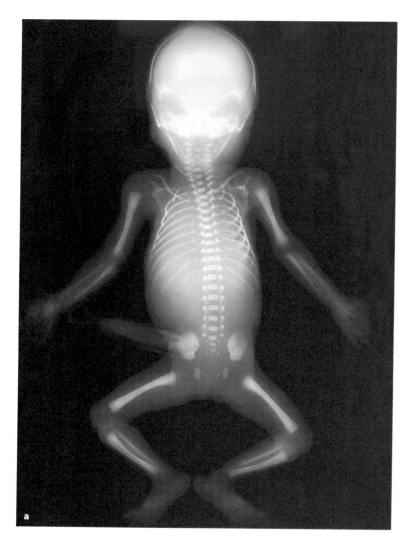

Fig. 1.13a, b. (Half original size) *Week 23.* Length of femur 39 mm (normal range 34–44 mm)
Milestone: Sternal ossification centers appear
Sternal ossification starts with the simultaneous appearance of ossifi-cation centers in the manubrium and corpus sterni. Pubic bones are clearly seen and the calcanei are ossified in approximately 50% of fetuses

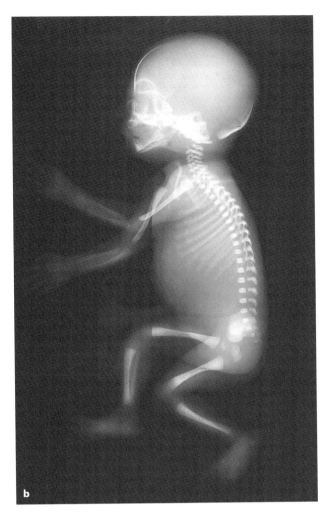

Fig. 1.13b

Femur

Table 1.1. Relation of diaphyseal length (mm) and gestational week in the femur (adapted from Merz 1988, with permission of the author)

mm	Gestational week			mm	Gestational week		
	5%	50%	95%		5%	50%	95%
10	12	13	14	45	24	26	27
11	12	13	14	46	24	26	27
12	12	13	15	47	24	26	28
13	13	14	15	48	25	27	28
14	13	14	15	49	25	27	29
15	13	14	16	50	26	27	29
16	14	15	16	51	26	28	30
17	14	15	16	52	26	28	30
18	14	15	17	53	27	29	30
19	15	16	17	54	27	29	31
20	15	16	18	55	28	29	31
21	15	17	18	56	28	30	32
22	16	17	18	57	28	30	32
23	16	17	19	58	29	31	32
24	16	18	19	59	29	31	33
25	17	18	19	60	30	31	33
26	17	18	20	61	30	32	34
27	17	19	20	62	30	32	34
28	18	19	20	63	31	33	35
29	18	19	21	64	31	33	35
30	18	20	21	65	32	34	36
31	19	20	22	66	32	34	36
32	19	20	22	67	32	34	36
33	19	21	22	68	33	35	37
34	20	21	23	69	33	35	37
35	20	22	23	70	34	36	38
36	20	22	24	71	34	36	38
37	21	22	24	72	35	37	39
38	21	23	24	73	35	37	39
39	21	23	25	74	36	38	40
40	22	23	25	75	36	38	40
41	22	24	25	76	36	39	41
42	23	24	26	77	37	39	41
43	23	25	26	78	37	40	42
44	23	25	27	79	37	40	42

Tibia

Table 1.2. Relation of diaphyseal length and gestational week in the tibia (adapted from Merz 1988, with permission of the author)

mm	Gestational week			mm	Gestational week		
	5%	50%	95%		5%	50%	95%
8	11	13	14	38	23	25	27
9	12	13	14	39	23	25	27
10	12	13	15	40	24	26	28
11	13	14	15	41	24	26	28
12	13	14	16	42	25	27	28
13	13	15	16	43	25	27	29
14	14	15	16	44	26	28	29
15	14	15	17	45	26	28	30
16	14	16	17	46	27	29	30
17	15	16	18	47	27	29	31
18	15	16	18	48	28	30	31
19	15	17	18	49	28	30	32
20	16	17	19	50	28	31	33
21	16	18	19	51	29	31	33
22	17	18	20	52	29	32	34
23	17	18	20	53	30	32	34
24	17	19	20	54	31	33	35
25	18	19	21	55	31	33	35
26	18	20	21	56	32	34	36
27	18	20	22	57	32	34	36
28	19	20	22	58	33	35	37
29	19	21	23	59	33	35	38
30	20	21	23	60	34	36	38
31	20	22	23	61	34	37	39
32	20	22	24	62	35	37	39
33	21	23	24	63	36	38	40
34	21	23	25	64	36	38	41
35	22	23	25	65	37	39	41
36	22	24	26	66	37	40	42
37	23	24	26	67	38	40	43

Humerus

Table 1.3. Relation of diaphyseal length and gestational week in the humerus (adapted from Merz 1988, with permission of the author)

mm	Gestational week			mm	Gestational week		
	5%	50%	95%		5%	50%	95%
9	11	13	14	39	23	25	26
10	12	13	14	40	23	26	27
11	12	13	15	41	23	25	27
12	12	14	15	42	24	26	28
13	13	14	16	43	24	26	28
14	13	14	16	44	25	27	29
15	13	15	16	45	25	27	29
16	14	15	17	46	26	28	30
17	14	16	17	47	26	28	30
18	14	16	17	48	27	29	31
19	15	16	18	49	27	29	31
20	15	17	18	50	28	30	32
21	16	17	19	51	28	30	32
22	16	18	19	62	29	31	33
23	16	18	19	53	29	31	34
24	17	18	20	54	30	32	34
25	17	19	20	55	30	32	35
26	17	19	21	56	31	33	35
27	18	19	21	57	31	34	36
28	18	20	22	58	32	34	36
29	19	20	22	59	32	35	37
30	19	21	22	60	33	36	38
31	19	21	23	61	34	36	38
32	20	22	23	62	34	36	39
33	20	22	24	63	35	37	39
34	21	22	24	64	35	38	40
35	21	23	25	65	36	38	41
36	21	23	25	66	37	39	41
37	22	24	26	67	37	40	42
38	22	24	26	68	38	40	43

Radius

Table 1.4. Relation of diaphyseal length and gestational week in the radius (adapted from Merz 1988, with permission of the author)

mm	Gestational week			mm	Gestational week		
	5%	50%	95%		5%	50%	95%
6	11	13	14	31	22	24	26
7	11	13	15	32	22	24	27
8	12	13	15	33	23	25	27
9	12	14	16	34	23	26	28
10	12	14	16	35	24	26	29
11	13	15	16	36	24	27	29
12	13	15	17	37	25	27	30
13	14	15	17	38	25	28	30
14	14	16	18	39	26	28	31
15	14	16	18	40	26	29	32
16	15	17	19	41	27	30	32
17	15	17	19	42	28	30	33
18	16	18	20	43	28	31	34
19	16	18	20	44	29	32	34
20	16	19	21	45	30	32	35
21	17	19	21	46	30	33	36
22	17	19	22	47	31	34	37
23	18	20	22	48	32	35	37
24	18	20	23	49	32	35	38
25	19	21	23	50	33	36	39
26	19	21	24	51	34	37	40
27	20	22	24	52	35	38	41
28	20	22	25	53	36	39	42
29	21	23	25	54	36	40	43
30	21	23	26	55	37	40	44

Ulna

Table 1.5. Relation of diaphyseal length and gestational week in the ulna (adapted from Merz 1988, with permission of the author)

mm	Gestational week			mm	Gestational week		
	5%	50%	95%		5%	50%	95%
7	11	13	14	35	22	24	26
8	12	13	14	36	22	24	26
9	12	13	15	37	23	25	27
10	12	14	15	38	23	25	27
11	13	14	16	39	24	26	28
12	13	15	16	40	24	26	28
13	13	15	16	41	25	27	29
14	14	15	17	42	25	27	29
15	14	16	17	43	26	28	30
16	15	16	17	44	26	28	30
17	15	16	18	45	27	29	31
18	15	17	18	46	27	29	31
19	16	17	19	47	28	30	32
20	16	18	19	48	28	30	33
21	16	18	19	49	29	31	33
22	17	18	20	50	29	32	34
23	17	19	20	51	30	32	34
24	17	19	21	52	31	33	35
25	18	19	21	53	31	34	36
26	18	20	22	54	32	34	36
27	19	20	22	55	33	35	37
28	19	21	22	56	33	36	38
29	19	21	23	57	34	36	39
30	20	22	23	58	35	37	39
31	20	22	24	59	36	38	40
32	21	22	24	60	36	39	41
33	21	23	25	61	37	40	42
34	21	23	25	62	38	40	43

2 Differential Diagnosis of Single Skeletal Defects

Introduction

This section focuses on the radiographic differential diagnosis of single defects of the fetal skeleton. Complying with the character of this book as a radiographic tool, the number of conditions in the differential lists has been limited in two ways:

1. The disorder should have at least one radiographic sign in addition to the key feature, thus allowing one to make a diagnosis or suspect a diagnosis by radiographic analysis alone. For instance, the combination of an amputated limb with anencephaly – both recognizable on a fetogram – leads to a diagnosis of the ADAM complex. On the other hand, isolated vertebral segmentation defects in the upper thoracic spine without additional radiographic findings are relatively unspecific and can be seen in a great number of disorders. As radiology does not help in the differential diagnostic process, these isolated defects have not been included.

2. The disorder should be relatively common, i.e., have an entry in the OMIM database. Isolated case reports without an OMIM number have not been included in the differential diagnostic lists. Comprehensive lists of all possible disorders associated with a given defect are available in databases such as POSSUM or the London dysmorphology database.

The radiodiagnostic process requires the complete and thorough analysis of the available radiographs. Form, size, position, proportions, structure, and maturational status of all skeletal elements must be scrutinized. Soft tissue changes must be recorded. A pattern of findings may emerge from which a key skeletal feature is selected. Consulting the subsection devoted to this key feature, a diagnosis may emerge from a match between the given and a listed pattern. The presence of widespread, often symmetric, skeletal abnormalities raises the possibility of a generalized skeletal dysplasia (see Chap. 3). Tables in the appendix simplify this approach.

References

Danks D, Bankier A (2001) Possum 5.6. Murdoch Children's Research Institute, Parkville, Victoria, Australia

Winter R, Baraitser M (2001) London dysmorphology database 3.0. Oxford University Press Electronic Publishing

Amelia – Amputation – Phocomelia

Definition:
– Amelia: no formation of extremity
– Amputation: transverse terminal defects of limb (Fig. 2.1)
– Phocomelia: band-like or segmental defects within a limb (Fig. 2.2)

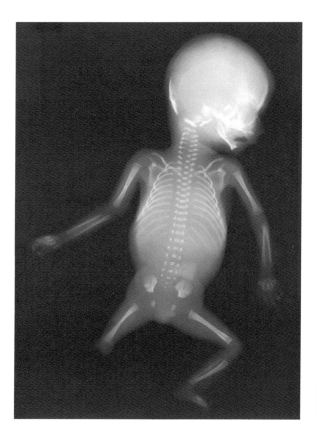

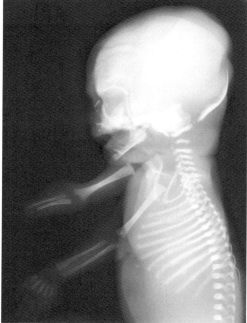

Fig. 2.1. *18th gestational week.* Amputation of the right shank in amniotic disruption sequence, otherwise normal skeleton

Fig. 2.2. *23rd gestational week.* Phocomelia of the left forearm with tiny fingers and a few dot-like phalangeal ossification centers

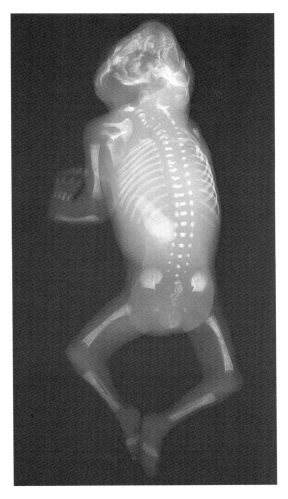

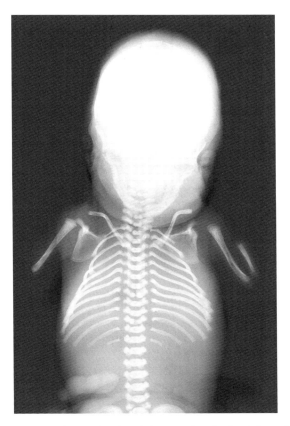

Fig. 2.3. *15th gestational week*. Amputation of the left arm in ADAM complex. Aplasia of the right radius and thumb; anencephaly, duplication of right scapula, hypoplastic clavicle

Fig. 2.4. *27th gestational week*. Asymmetric reduction defects of the forearms in oromandibular-limb hypogenesis syndrome. Hypoplasia of humeri. Sagittal clefts of the vertebral bodies of D8 and D11. Thirteen pairs of ribs

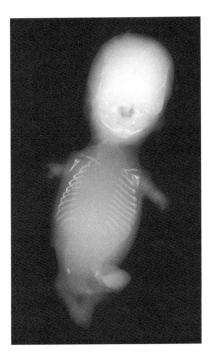

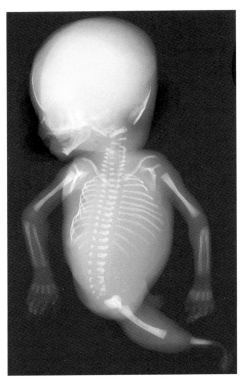

Fig. 2.5. *10th gestational week*. Short limbs. Roberts syndrome. Absent ossification of most tubular bones and age related absent ossification of the vertebrae

Fig. 2.6. *19th gestational week*. Monopodic sirenomelia. Pelvic fusion, sagittal cleft defects of the thoracic vertebral bodies. Accessory rib on the right at L1

Diagnosis	Accessory radiological findings in the fetus
Acrofacial dysostosis, type Rodriguez [1] MIM 201170	Phocomelia of arms, defective ulnar ray, short humerus and fibula, hypoplastic scapula
Amelia, autosomal recessive [2] MIM 601360	Amelia of upper limbs and terminal transverse defect through femora, micrognathia
Amnion disruption sequence ADAM complex (*Amniotic Deformity, Adhesions, Mutilations*); Fig. 2.3 Limb-body wall complex [3] MIM 217100	Terminal limb defects, constriction bands, distal lymphedema, different degree of mutilations, craniofacial clefts, ectopia cordis, cephalocele/anencephaly, body wall defects
Diabetic embryopathy [4]	Caudal regression, segmentation defects of the spine, defects of ulna and tibia, femoral aplasia
DK phocomelia [5] Phocomelia-encephalocele-thrombocytopenia-urogenital malformation von Voss-Cherstvoy syndrome MIM 223340	Microcephaly; absent or hypoplastic humerus, radius, ulna, metacarpals, thumb; oligodactyly; syndactyly of fingers; other features: genitourinary and cardiac anomalies, platelet abnormalities
Oromandibula-limb hypogenesis syndromes (incl. Hanhart syndrome) [6]; MIM 103300 Fig. 2.4	Nearly symmetric terminal limb reduction anomalies, micrognathia, hypoglossia

Diagnosis	Accessory radiological findings in the fetus
Roberts (pseudothalidomide) syndrome [7]; MIM 268300 Fig. 2.5	Tetraphocomelia, severe limb shortening, radial defects, oligodactyly, nuchal cystic hygroma, cleft palate, sometimes craniostenosis
Schinzel phocomelia [8] MIM 268300 May be the same as Al-Awadi/Raas-Rothschild syndrome Limb/pelvis hypoplasia/aplasia syndrome [9] MIM 276820	Variable and possibly asymmetric lower limb deficiency including primarily femur, tibia and fibula; absent toes; upper limb defects including absent/hypoplastic radius, ulna; radio-humeral synostosis; abscence of carpals, metacarpals, and phalanges; hypoplastic pelvis including irregular pubis, ischium; hip dislocation; thoracic involvement including wide or fused ribs, pectus carinatum
Sirenomelia [10] (part of caudal regression sequence); MIM 182940 Fig. 2.6	Fusion and varying degrees of hypoplasia of lower extremities; pelvic bone fusion; fusion of femurs, sometimes both tibiae and fibulae rotated by 180 degrees (see Fig. 2.37), spinal segmentation anomalies, bladder exstrophy, meningomyelocele, hypoplastic/absent radius
Splenogonadal fusion – limb defects [11] MIM 183300	Micrognathia, caudal regression, spinal dysraphism, transverse limb reduction with or without digits
Tetraamelia with multiple malformations [12] MIM 301090	Anencephalus, hydrocephalus, facial cleft, segmentation defects of spine, aplasia of pelvic bones, severe reduction defects of upper and lower limbs, no digits; other defect: anal atresia
Thalidomide embryopathy [13]	Amelia, proximal phocomelia, fingers present, often attached directly to the shoulders
Thrombocytopenia-absent radius (TAR) syndrome (severe form) [14] MIM 274000	Bilateral severe phocomelia of the upper limbs with hands, including thumbs, attached to the shoulders

References

1. Rodriguez JI, Palacios J, Urioste M (1992) Acrofacial dysostosis syndromes (letter). Am J Med Genet 42:851–852
2. Michaud J, Filiatrault D, Dallaire L, Lambert M (1995) New autosomal recessive form of amelia. Am J Med Genet 56:164–167
3. Higginbottom MC, Jones KL, Hall BD (1979) The amniotic band disruption complex: timing of amniotic rupture and variable spectra of consequent defects. J Pediatr 95:544–549
4. Dunn V, Nixon GW, Jaffe RB, Condon VR (1981) Infants of diabetic mothers: radiographic manifestations. AJR 137:123–128
5. Cherstvoy E, Lazjuk G, Lurie I et al (1980) Syndrome of multiple congenital malformations including phocomelia, thrombocytopenia, encephalocele and urogenital abnormalities. Lancet 2:485
6. Chicarilli ZN, Polayes IM (1985) Oromandibular limb hypogenesis syndromes. Plast Reconstr Surg 76:13–24
7. Van den Berg DJ, Francke U (1993) Roberts syndrome: a review of 100 cases and a new rating system for severity. Am J Med Genet 47:1104–1123
8. Lurie IW, Wulfsberg EA (1993) On the nosology of the "Schinzel-phocomelia" and "Al-Awadi/Raas-Rothschild" syndromes (letter). Am J Med Genet 47:1234

9. Raas-Rothschild A, Goodman RM, Meyer S et al (1988) Pathological features and prenatal diagnosis in the newly-recognized limb/pelvis-hypoplasia/aplasia syndrome. J Med Genet 25:687–697
10. Currarino G, Weinberg A (1991) From small pelvic outlet syndrome to sirenomelia. Pediatr Pathol 11:195–210
11. Gouw ASH, Elema JD, Bink-Boelkens MTE et al (1985) The spectrum of splenogonadal fusion. Case report and review of 84 reported cases. Eur J Pediatr 144:316–323
12. Zimmer EZ, Taub E, Sova Y, Divon MY, Pery M, Peretz BA (1985) Tetra-amelia with multiple malformations in six male fetuses of one kindred. Eur J Pediatr 144:412–414
13. Newman CGH (1985) Teratogen update: clinical aspects of thalidomide embryopathy – a continuing preoccupation. Teratology 32:133–144
14. Delooz J, Moerman P, van den Berghe K, Fryns JP (1992) Tetraphocomelia and bilateral femorotibial synostosis. A severe variant of the thrombocytopenia-absent radii (TAR) syndrome? Genet Counsel 3:91–93

Aplasia/Hypoplasia of Thumb and Radius [1]

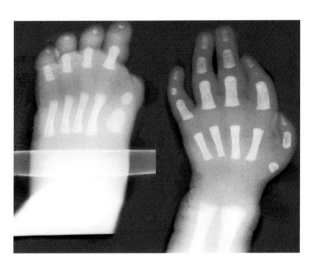

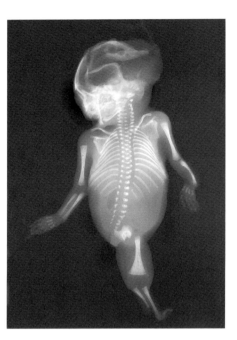

Fig. 2.7. *Newborn.* Isolated hypoplasia of metacarpal and phalanges of thumb; Brachymesophalangy II and V. Hypoplasia of metatarsal and aplasia of terminal phalanx of hallux in fibrodysplasia ossificans progressiva

Fig. 2.8. *19th gestational week.* Dipodic sirenomelia. Aplasia of the thumb in both hands, aplasia of the left radius, 13 pairs of ribs, and accessory cervical ribs. Fusion of femora, aplasia of fibulae, hypoplastic tibiae.(Postmortem laceration of the neurocranium)

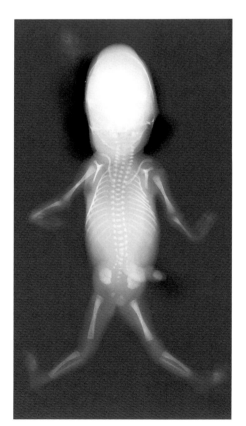

Fig. 2.9. *18th gestational week.* Aplasia of radius on both sides in VACTERL association. Segmentation defects of the lumbar and sacral vertebrae. Vertebral fusion. Hyperextended knees are a sequelae of intrauterine malposition due to anhydramnios. Asymmetric shape and narrow position of the ischia suggest an underlying urethral pathology – see "Pelvic-Sacral Abnormalities". Other findings: esophageal atresia Vogt II; urethral atresia; multicystic, dysplastic horseshoe kidney

Diagnosis	Accessory radiological findings in the fetus
Acrofacial dysostosis, type Rodriguez [2] MIM 263750	Micrognathia, forearm anomalies mostly on the radial side, short forearm, radio-ulnar synostosis, preaxial polydactyly, fibular hypoplasia
Amnion disruption sequence ADAM complex (Amniotic Deformity, Adhesions, Mutilations) [3] Limb-body wall complex MIM 217100	Terminal limb defects, constriction bands, distal lymphedema, different degree of mutilations, craniofacial clefts, ectopia cordis, cephalocele/anencephaly, body wall defects
Baller-Gerold Syndrome [4] MIM 218600	Asymmetric radial defect; shortened, bowed ulna; variable premature craniosynostosis; preferable coronal suture
Brachmann-de Lange Syndrome [5] MIM 122470	Primordial dwarfism; hand with ray reduction, mainly ulnar aplasia
Chromosome abnormality Trisomy 18 (Edward Syndrome) [6]	Slender ribs (11 pairs), vertical iliac bones, limb reduction, radioulnar synostosis, rocker-bottom foot, typical flexion deformity of fingers and overlapping of 2nd finger (see Fig. 2.40), omphalocele
Chromosome 13 q syndrome [7]; see Fig. 2.31	Growth retardation, absent thumb, proximal synostosis of metacarpals/tarsals 4 and 5
Fanconi pancytopenia [1] MIM 227650	Range from aplastic thumb to duplication
Thrombocytopenia-absent radius (TAR) syndrome [1] MIM 274000	Bilateral aplasia of radius but present thumbs
Fetal valproate syndrome [8, 9]	Prominent metopic ridge, bifrontal narrowing, clinodactyly, distal phalangeal hypoplasia, absent or hypoplastic radius, absent or hypoplastic thumb, talipes equinovarus
Fibrodysplasia ossificans progressiva [10]; MIM 135100 Fig. 2.7	Isolated aplasia/hypoplasia of metacarpal and phalanges of thumb and metatarsal and phalanges of hallux
Fryns syndrome – acral defects [11] MIM 229850	Distal ray hypoplasia; other finding: diaphragmatic hernia
Goldenhar syndrome (oculo-auriculo-vertebral dysplasia) [12]; MIM 164210 see Fig. 2.32	Sporadic, unilateral malformation syndrome of the first and second branchial arches (hypoplastic mandible and maxilla), vertebral anomalies, radial hypoplasia
Holt-Oram (cardiomelic) syndrome [1] MIM 142900	Triphalangeal thumb, radio-ulnar synostosis, absent radius, absent ulna, hypoplastic humerus
Mesomelic dysplasias [13]; see p. 155 ff	Symmetric mesomelic (forearm, shank) shortening of the extremities, different types
MURCS association [14]; MIM 601076 see Fig. 2.34	Acronym of associated malformations: *Mu*llerian duct aplasia/hypoplasia, *r*enal aplasia/ectopia, *c*ervical *s*omite (*s*pinal) dysplasia; upper limb defects
Nager acrofacial dysostosis [15] MIM 154400	Forearm anomalies, aplasia/hypoplasia on the radial side, radio-ulnar synostosis, micrognathia
Poland syndrome [16] MIM 173800	Different degrees of finger and radius defects, vertebral anomalies; other defect: aplasia of pectoralis muscle

Diagnosis	Accessory radiological findings in the fetus
Roberts (pseudothalidomide) syndrome [17]; MIM 268300 see Fig. 2.5	Tetraphocomelia, severe limb shortening, radial and ulnar defects, oligodactyly, nuchal cystic hygroma, sometimes craniostenosis
Sirenomelia [18] (part of caudal regression sequence); MIM 182940 Fig. 2.8	Fusion and varying degrees of hypoplasia of lower extremities, pelvic bone fusion, fusion of femurs; overlap with VACTERL association
VACTERL Association [1]; MIM 192350 Fig. 2.9	Acronym of associated malformations: Vertebral malsegmentation, anal atresia, cardiac malformation, tracheoesophageal fistula, esophageal atresia, radial/renal anomalies, limb anomalies (ray defects such as hypoplasia of fibula, tibia, aplasia of metatarsals, oligo-/preaxial polydactyly of fingers)

In cases with isolated aplasia of the radius or radial ray, no other radiological apparent defects are found.

References

1. Cox H, Viljoen DL, Versfeld G, Beighton P (1989) Radial ray defects and associated anomalies. Clin Genet 35:322–330
2. Rodriguez JI, Palacios J, Urioste M (1990) New acrofacial dysostosis syndrome in 3 sibs. Am J Med Genet 35:484–489
3. Higginbottom MC, Jones KL, Hall BD (1979) The amniotic band disruption complex: timing of amniotic rupture and variable spectra of consequent defects. J Pediatr 95:544–549
4. Boudreaux JM, Colon MA, Lorusso GD et al (1990) Baller-Gerold syndrome: an 11th case of craniosynostosis and radial aplasia. Am J Med Genet 37:447–450
5. Braddock SR, Lachman RS, Stoppenhagen CC et al (1993) Radiological al features in Brachmann-de Lange syndrome. Am J Med Genet 47:1006–1013
6. Schinzel A (1979) Autosomale Chromosomenaberrationen. Arch Genet (Zur) 52:1–204
7. Sparkes RS, Carrel RE, Wright SW (1967) Absent thumbs with a ring D2 chromosome; a new deletion syndrome. Am J Hum Genet 19:644–654
8. Robert E, Guibaud P (1982) Maternal valproic acid and congenital neural tube defects. Lancet 2:937
9. Sharony R, Garber A, Viskochil D et al (1993) Preaxial ray reduction defects as part of valproic acid embryofetopathy. Prenatal Diag 13:909–918
10. Schroeder H Jr, Zasloff M (1980) The hand and foot malformations in fibrodysplasia ossificans progressiva. Johns Hopkins Med J 147:73–78
11. Cunniff C, Jones KL, Saal HM, Stern HJ (1990) Fryns syndrome: an autosomal recessive disorder associated with craniofacial anomalies, diaphragmatic hernia, and distal digital hypoplasia. Pediatrics 85:499–504
12. Coccaro PJ, Becker MH, Converse JM (1975) Clinical and radiographic variations in hemifacial microsomia. BDOAS 11:314–324
13. Kaitila II, Leisti T, Rimoin CL (1976) Mesomelic skeletal dysplasias. Clin Orthoped 114:94–106
14. Greene RA, Bloch MJ, Shuff DS, Iozzo RV (1986) MURCS association with additional congenital anomalies. Hum Pathol 17:88–91
15. Pfeiffer RA, Stoess H (1983) Acrofacial dysostosis (Nager syndrome): synopsis and report of a new case. Am J Med Genet 15:255–260
16. Lord MJ, Laurenzano KR, Hartmann RW Jr (1990) Poland's syndrome. Clin Pediatr 29:606–609
17. Van den Berg DJ, Francke U (1993) Roberts syndrome: a review of 100 cases and a new rating system for severity. Am J Med Genet 47:1104–1123
18. Currarino G, Weinberg A (1991) From small pelvic outlet syndrome to sirenomelia. Pediatr Pathol 11:195–210

Readers' Notes:

Radio-ulnar Synostosis (Fig. 2.10)

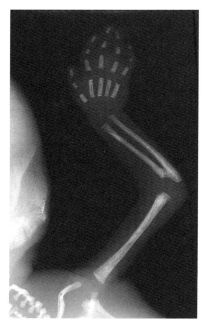

Fig. 2.10. *19th gestational week.* Radioulnar synostosis in Triploidy. Bone bridge between the proximal parts of radius and ulna

Diagnosis	Accessory radiological findings in the fetus
Cenani-Lenz syndrome [1] MIM 212780	Variable degree of radio-ulnar synostosis up to complete fusion; extensive phalangeal synostosis and proximal metacarpal fusion; oligodactyly; thoracic hemivertebrae
Cloverleaf skull – limb anomaly, type Holtermüller-Wiedemann [2] MIM 148800	Trilobed skull deformity (congenital cranial synostosis), ankylosis of elbow
Chromosome abnormality Trisomy 18 [3]	Slender ribs (11 pairs), vertical iliac bones, rocker-bottom foot, hypoplasia of first metacarpal, typical flexion deformities and overlapping 2nd finger (see Fig. 2.40), omphalocele, limb reduction
Chromosome abnormality Klinefelter syndrome [4]	No specific radiologic signs in the fetus
Fetal alcohol syndrome [5]	Intrauterine growth retardation, vertebral segmentation defects, Klippel-Feil syndrome, reduction deformity of upper extremities, hypoplasia/ aplasia of ulna, tetradactyly; clubfoot
Holt-Oram syndrome (cardiomelic syndrome) [6] MIM 142900	Triphalangeal thumb, hypoplastic/absent radius, hypoplastic/absent ulna, hypoplastic humerus
Nager acrofacial dysostosis [7] MIM 154400	Forearm anomalies: aplasia/hypoplasia on the radial side, radio-ulnar synostosis; micrognathia
Radio-ulnar synostosis, autosomal dominant [8] MIM 179300	Bilateral or single-sided proximal synostosis

References

1. Pfeiffer RA, Meisel-Stosiek M (1982) Present nosology of the Cenani-Lenz type of syndactyly. Clin Genet 21:74–79
2. Holtermüller K, Wiedemann H-R (1960) Kleeblattschädel Syndrom. Med Monatsschr 14:439–446
3. Franceschini P, Fabris C, Ponzone A et al (1974) Skeletal alterations in Edwards' disease (trisomy 18 syndrome). Ann Radiol (Paris) 17:361–367
4. Jancu J (1971) Radioulnar synostosis in sex chromosome abnormalities. Am J Dis Child 122:10–11
5. Herrmann J, Pallister PD, Opitz JM (1980) Tetraectrodactyly, and other skeletal manifestations in the fetal alcohol syndrome. Eur J Pediatr 133:221–226
6. Smith AT, Sack GH, Taylor GJ (1979) Holt-Oram syndrome. J Pediatr 95:538–543
7. Pfeiffer RA, Stoess H (1983) Acrofacial dysostosis (Nager syndrome): synopsis and report of a new case. Am J Med Genet 15:255–260
8. Rizzo R, Pavone V, Corsello G, Sorge G, Neri G, Opitz JM (1997) Autosomal dominant and sporadic Radio-ulnar synostosis. Am J Med Genet 68:127–134

Ulna: Aplasia, Hypoplasia

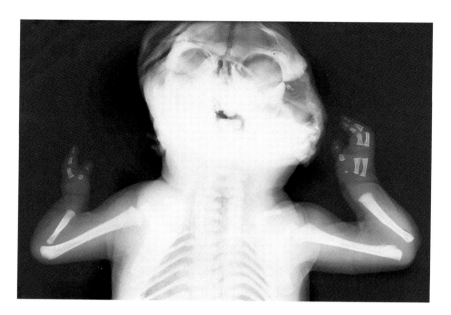

Fig. 2.11. *33rd gestational week.* Complex tubular bone aplasia/hypoplasia in Brachmann-De Lange syndrome: bilateral aplasia of the ulna and ulnar rays of the hands, aplasia of the middle finger and proximal phalanx of the thumb on the right side. Hypoplastic radii. Luxation of the left humeroradial joint

Diagnosis	Accessory radiological findings in the fetus
Acrofacial dysostosis with post-axial defects [1] MIM 263750	Different degrees of postaxial hypoplasia in all four limbs, shortened forearm
Acrofacial dysostosis, type Rodriguez [2] MIM 263750	Micrognathia, forearm anomalies mostly on the radial side, short forearm, radio-ulnar synostosis, preaxial polydactyly, fibular hypoplasia
Brachmann-de Lange syndrome [3]; MIM 122470 Fig. 2.11	Variable reduction deficiency of upper limb, including ulna, humerus, radius, carpals; ectrodactyly
Femur-fibula-ulna complex (FFU syndrome) [4] MIM 228200	Asymmetric hypoplasia/aplasia of femur, fibula, humerus, ulna; humero-ulnar/-radial synostosis; oligodactyly
Fetal alcohol syndrome [5]	Intrauterine growth retardation, vertebral segmentation defects, Klippel-Feil syndrome, reduction deformity of upper extremities, hypoplasia/aplasia of ulna, radio-ulnar synostosis, tetradactyly, clubfoot
Grebe syndrome [6, 7] and related osteochondrodysplasias; see p. 159 MIM 200700	Dislocated radial heads, aplasia/hypoplasia of ulna, radius, femur; absent or hypoplastic proximal and middle phalanges; syndactyly; absent or hypoplastic metacarpals; absent or hypoplastic carpals; carpal fusion; very short tubular long bones (lower limbs more severe than upper limbs), hypoplastic tarsals, short and broad metatarsals
Holt-Oram-Syndrome (cardiomelic syndrome) [8] MIM 142900	Asymmetric aplasia of radius, triphalangeal thumb, hypoplasia of humerus
Lethal osteochondrodysplasias [9]; see p. 150	For example, atelosteogenesis II (de la Chapelle dysplasia)

Diagnosis	Accessory radiological findings in the fetus
Mesomelic dysplasias [10]; see p. 155 ff	Severe mesomelic (i.e., forearm, shank) shortening of the extremities, different types
Neu-Laxova syndrome [11] MIM 256520	Severe microcephaly, hypoplasia of radius/ulna, post-axial oligodactyly
Neurofibromatosis 1 [12] MIM 162200	Pseudarthrosis; pathologic fracture of the diaphysis due to focal fibrous dysplasia; most often in the tibia
Roberts (pseudothalidomide) syndrome [13]; see Fig. 2.5 MIM 268300	Tetraphocomelia, severe limb shortening, radial defects, oligodactyly, nuchal cystic hygroma, sometimes cranio-stenosis
Thrombocytopenia-absent radius (TAR) syndrome [14] MIM 274000	Bilateral aplasia of radius but present thumbs
Ulnar-mammary syndrome type Pallister [15] MIM 181450	Ulnar ray deficiency, aplasia of phalanges, bowed radius, hypoplasia of humerus; other: anal atresia/stenosis
Weyers syndrome of deficiency of ulnar and fibular rays [16] MIM 193530	Hypoplasia of ulna and fingers, split hand, absent clavicles, cleft palate; see also "Fibula: Aplasia. Hypoplasia"

References

1. Fryns JP, van den Berghe H (1988) Acrofacial dysostosis with postaxial limb deficiency. Am J Med Genet 29:205–208
2. Rodriguez JI, Palacios J, Urioste M (1990) New acrofacial dysostosis syndrome in 3 sibs. Am J Med Genet 35:484–489
3. Braddock SR, Lachman RS, Stoppenhagen CC et al (1993) Radiological al features in Brachmann-de Lange syndrome. Am J Med Genet 47:1006–1013
4. Lenz W, Zygulska M, Horst J (1993) FFU complex: an analysis of 491 cases. Hum Genet 91:347–356
5. Herrmann J, Pallister PD, Opitz JM (1980) Tetraectrodactyly, and other skeletal manifestations in the fetal alcohol syndrome. Eur J Pediatr 133:221–226
6. Grebe H (1952) Die Achondrogenesis: ein einfach rezessives Erbmerkmal. Folia Hered Path 2:23–28
7. Costa T, Ramsby G, Cassia F et al (1998) Grebe syndrome: clinical and radiographic findings in affected individuals and heterozygous carriers. Am J Med Genet 75:523–529
8. Smith AT, Sack GH, Taylor GJ (1979) Holt-Oram syndrome. J Pediatr 95:538–543
9. Spranger J, Maroteaux P (1990) The lethal chondrodysplasias. Adv Hum Genet 19:1–103
10. Kaitila II, Leisti T, Rimoin CL (1976) Mesomelic skeletal dysplasias. Clin Orthoped 114:94–106
11. Rouzbahani L (1995) New manifestations in an infant with Neu Laxova syndrome (letter). Am J Med Genet 56:239–240
12. Bell DF (1989) Congenital forearm pseudarthrosis: report of six cases and review of the literature. J Pediatr Orthop 9:438–443
13. Van den Berg DJ, Francke U (1993) Roberts syndrome: a review of 100 cases and a new rating system for severity. Am J Med Genet 47:1104–1123
14. Botto LD, Khoury MJ, Mastroiacovo P et al (1997) The spectrum of congenital anomalies of the VATER association: an international study. Am J Med Genet 71:8–16
15. Schinzel A(1987) Ulnar-mammary syndrome. J Med Genet 24:778–781
16. Weyers H (1957) Das Oligodaktylie Syndrom des Menschen und seine parallele Mutation bei der Hausmaus (Oligodactylia syndrome in humans and its parallel mutation in the house mouse). Ann Paediatr (Basel) 189:351–370

Humerus: Aplasia, Hypoplasia

Diagnosis	Accessory radiological findings in the fetus
Acrofacial dysostosis, type Rodriguez [1] MIM 201170	Phocomelia of arms, defective ulnar ray, short humerus and fibula, hypoplastic scapula
Atelosteogenesis I [2–4] and related osteochondrodysplasias; see p. 148 MIM 108720, 108721, 112310	Hypoplastic vertebral bodies, especially of cervical and thoracic spine; hypoplastic and tapered (distal) humerus and femur; bowed radius, ulna and tibia; absent or hypoplastic fibula; absent or hypo-ossified metacarpals and phalanges
Brachmann-de Lange syndrome [5]; see Fig. 2.11 MIM 122470	Variable reduction deficiency of upper limb, including ulna, humerus, radius, carpals; ectrodactyly
CHILD syndrome [6] (Congenital hemidysplasia, ichthyosiform erythroderma, limb defects) MIM 308050	Unilateral hypoplasia of limb(s) including absent or hypoplastic scapula, humerus, radius, ulna, femur, tibia, fibula; joint contracture or pterygium; punctate epiphyseal calcification; other features: congenital ichthyosiform erythroderma ipsilateral to limb deficiency, visceral anomalies
Chondrodysplasia punctata, rhizomelic type [7, 8]; see p. 142 MIM 215100	Punctate calcifications primarily around the ends of the long bones, hypoplasia of humerus and femur, wide or splayed metaphyses, platyspondyly
Chondrodysplasia punctata, tibia-metacarpal type [9]; MIM 118651	Stippling of sacrum and carpals; dislocation of hip, knee, elbow; short tibia, femur, metacarpals, phalanges; asymmetry
DK phocomelia [10] Phocomelia-encephalocele-thrombocytopenia-urogenital malformation von Voss-Cherstvoy syndrome MIM 223340	Microcephaly; absent or hypoplastic humerus, radius, ulna, metacarpals, thumb; oligodactyly; syndactyly of fingers; other features: genitourinary, cardiac anomalies, platelet abnormalities
Femur-fibula-ulna complex (FFU syndrome) [11] MIM 228200	Asymmetric hypoplasia/aplasia of femur, fibula, humerus, ulna; humero-ulnar/-radial synostosis; oligodactyly
Fetal thalidomide [12]	Amelia; proximal phocomelia; fingers present, often attached direct to the shoulders
Fetal valproate syndrome [13, 14]	Prominent metopic ridge, bifrontal narrowing, clinodactyly, distal phalangeal hypoplasia, absent or hypoplastic radius, absent or hypoplastic thumb, talipes equinovarus
Holt-Oram syndrome [15, 16] Cardiomelic syndrome MIM 142900	Absent or hypoplastic humerus, radius, ulna, first metacarpal, thumb; triphalangeal thumb; absent or hypoplastic carpals; delayed ossification or fusion of carpals; other polydactyly; radioulnar synostosis; hypoplasia of the clavicle, scapula; Sprengel anomaly; pectus excavatum or carinatum; rib hypoplasia or fusion; vertebral fusion or hemivertebra, scoliosis; other anomalies: cardiac defects (secundum-type atrial septal defect most commonly)

Diagnosis	Accessory radiological findings in the fetus
Omodysplasia [17–19]; see p. 152￼ MIM 164745, 251455	Rhizomelia of upper limbs by distal hypoplasia of humeri, milder such involvement of lower limbs; dislocation of radial heads
Oromandibular–limb hypogenesis syndromes; see Fig. 2.20 Aglossia-adactylia, hypoglossia-hypodactylia Hanhart syndrome [20, 21] MIM 103300	Asymmetric, variably absent or hypoplastic humerus, radius, ulna, carpals, metacarpals, femur, tibia, fibula, tarsals, metatarsals; oligodactyly; syndactyly; microretrognathia; aplasia/hypoplasia of tongue
Thrombocytopenia-absent radius (TAR) syndrome (severe form) [22] MIM 274000	Bilateral severe phocomelia of the upper limbs with hands attached to the shoulders, thumbs present
Ulnar-mammary syndrome type Pallister [23] MIM 181450	Ulnar ray deficiency; aplasia of phalanges; bowed radius; hypoplasia of humerus; other: anal atresia/stenosis

References

1. Rodriguez JI, Palacios J, Urioste M (1992) Acrofacial dysostosis syndromes (letter). Am J Med Genet 42:851–852
2. Sillence DO, Worthington SD, Dixon J, Osborn R, Kozlowski K (1997) Atelosteogenesis syndromes: a review with comments on their pathogenesis. Pediatr Radiol 27:388–396
3. Hunter AGW, Carpenter BF (1991) Atelosteogenesis I and boomerang dysplasia: a question of nosology. Clin Genet 39:471–480
4. Winship I, Cremin B, Beighton P (1990) Boomerang dysplasia. Am J Med Genet 36:440–443
5. Braddock SR, Lachman RS, Stoppenhagen CC et al (1993) Radiological al features in Brachmann-de Lange syndrome. Am J Med Genet 47:1006–1013
6. Happle R, Koch H, Lenz W (1980) The CHILD syndrome: congenital hemidysplasia with ichthyosiform erythroderma and limb defects. Eur J Pediatr 134:27–33
7. Gilbert EF, lopitz JM, Spranger JW et al (1976) Chondrodysplasia punctata, rhizomelic form: pathological and radiologic studies in three infants. Eur J Pediatr 123:89–109
8. Poulos A, Sheffield L, Sharp P et al (1988) Rhizomelic chondrodysplasia punctata: clinical, pathologic and biochemical findings in two patients. J Pediatr 113:685–690
9. Rittler M, Menger H, Spranger J (1990) Chondrodysplasia punctata, tibia-metacarpal (MT) type. Am J Med Genet 37:200–208
10. Cherstvoy E, Lazjuk G, Lurie I et al (1980) Syndrome of multiple congenital malformations including phocomelia, thrombocytopenia, encephalocele and urogenital abnormalities Lancet 2:485
11. Lenz W, Zygulska M, Horst J (1993) FFU complex: an analysis of 491 cases. Hum Genet 91:347–356

12. Newman CGH (1985) Teratogen update: clinical aspects of thalidomide embryopathy – a continuing preoccupation. Teratology 32:133–144
13. Robert E, Guibaud P (1982) Maternal valproic acid and congenital neural tube defects. Lancet 2:937
14. Sharony R, Garber A, Viskochil D et al (1993) Preaxial ray reduction defects as part of valproic acid embryofetopathy. Prenatal Diag 13:909–918
15. Holt M, Oram S (1960) Familial heart disease with skeletal malformations. Br Heart J 22:236–242
16. Poznanski AK, Gall JC Jr, Stern AM (1970) Skeletal manifestations of the Holt-Oram syndrome. Radiology 94:45–53
17. Maroteaux P, Sauvegrain J, Chrispin A, Farriaux JP (1989) Omodysplasia. Am J Med Genet 32:371–375
18. Borochowitz Z, Barak M, Hershkowitz S (1991) Familial congenital micromelic dysplasia with dislocation of radius and distinct face: a new skeletal dysplasia syndrome. Am J Med Genet 39:91–96
19. Borochowitz Z, Barak M, Hershkowitz S (1995) Nosology of omodysplasia (letter). Am J Med Genet 58:377
20. Hall BD (1971) Aglossia-adactylia. Birth Defects Orig Artic Ser 7:233–236
21. Kelln EE, Bennet CG, Klingberg WG (1968) Aglossia-adactylia syndrome. Am J Dis Child 116:549–552
22. Delooz J, Moerman P, van den Berghe K, Fryns JP (1992) Tetraphocomelia and bilateral femorotibial synostosis. A severe variant of the thrombocytopenia-absent radii (TAR) syndrome? Genet Counsel 3:91–93
23. Schinzel A (1987) Ulnar-mammary syndrome. J Med Genet 24:778–781

Tibia: Aplasia, Hypoplasia

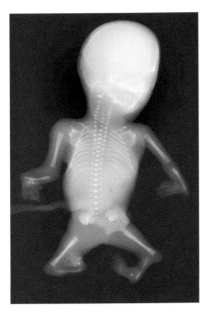

Fig. 2.12. *18th gestational week.* Aplasia of both radii and tibiae in Trisomy 18. Aplasia of the first ray of the left hand and foot. Punctate calcifications in the calcaneus. 11 pairs of slender ribs. (Note retarded maturation!)

Diagnosis	Accessory radiological findings in the fetus
Amniotic band disruption sequence ADAM complex (Amniotic Deformity, Adhesions, Mutilations) Limb-body wall complex [1]; see Fig. 2.24 MIM 217100	Usually asymmetric transverse terminal limb reductions/amputations and variable terminal syndactyly/pseudosyndactyly; sometimes also oligodactyly, hypoplasia of long bones, craniofacial and ventral wall disruption
Chondrodysplasia punctata, tibia-metacarpal type [2]; MIM 118651	Stippling of sacrum and carpals; dislocation of hip, knee, elbow; short tibia and femur; short metacarpals and phalanges; asymmetry
Chromosome abnormality Trisomy 18 [3]; Fig. 2.12	In rare cases tibial aplasia is present; for Trisomy 18 see "Aplasia, Hypoplasia of Thumb and Radius"
Grebe syndrome [4]; see p. 159 MIM 200700	Severe, proportionate shortening of extremities, mild shortening of trunk, absent proximal phalanges, distal phalanges always present, oligo/polydactyly
Mesomelic dysplasias [5]; see p. 155 ff	Different types and degree of mesomelic shortening of the extremities combined with or without phalangeal involvement.
Mesomelic dwarfism of hypoplastic tibia-radius type [6] MIM 156230	Isolated bilateral shortening of radius and tibia
Neurofibromatosis 1 [7] MIM 162200	Tibial pseudarthrosis; pathologic fracture of the diaphysis due to focal fibroma; rare in other long bones

Diagnosis	Accessory radiological findings in the fetus
Split hand/foot, tibial defect [8] MIM 119100	Split hand and/or foot; hypoplasia of ulna, femur; bifurcation of distal femur; postaxial polydactyly
Tibial hemimelia [9] MIM 275220	Isolated aplasia of the tibia, clubfoot
Tibial hypoplasia, polydactyly and triphalangeal thumb (Werner syndrome) [10] MIM 188770	Triphalangeal thumb, (multiple) preaxial polydactyly of feet, polydactyly of hands, radio-ulnar synostosis In rare cases tibial aplasia is present
VACTERL association	For VACTERL association see "Aplasia, Hypoplasia of Thumb and Radius"

References

1. Keeling JW, Kjaer I (1994) Diagnostic distinction between anencephaly and amnion rupture sequence based on skeletal analysis. J Med Gent 31:823–829
2. Rittler M, Menger H, Spranger J (1990) Chondrodysplasia punctata, tibia-metacarpal (MT) type. Am J Med Genet 37:200–208
3. Christianson AL, Nelson MM (1984) Four cases of trisomy 18 syndrome with limb reduction malformations. J Med Genet 21:293–297
4. Romeo G, Zonana J, Rimoin DL, Lachman RS, Scott C, Kaveggia EG, Spranger JW, Opitz JM (1977) Heterogeneity of nonlethal severe short-limbed dwarfism. J Pediatr 91:918–923
5. Kaitila II, Leisti T, Rimoin CL (1976) Mesomelic skeletal dysplasias. Clin Orthop 114:94–106
6. Leroy JG, de Vos J, Timmermans J (1975) Dominant mesomelic dwarfism of the hypoplastic tibia, radius type. Clin Genet 7:280–286
7. Boero S, Catagni M, Donzelli O, Facchini R, Frediani PV (1997) Congenital pseudarthrosis of the tibia associated with neurofibromatosis-1: treatment with Illizarov's device. J Pediatr Orthop 17:675–685
8. Majewski F, Kuster W, ter Haar B et al (1985) Aplasia of tibia with split-hand/split-foot deformity. Report of six families with 35 cases and considerations about variability and penetrance. Hum Genet 70:136–147
9. Schroer RJ, Meyer LC (1983) Autosomal dominant tibial hypoplasia-aplasia. Proc Gr Genet Center 2:27–31
10. Canun S, Lomeli RM, Martinez y Martinez R et al (1984) Absent tibiae, triphalangeal thumbs and polydactyly: description of a family and prenatal diagnosis. Clin Genet 25:182–186

Fibula: Aplasia, Hypoplasia

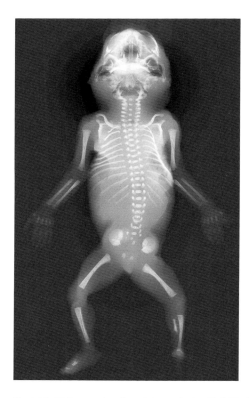

Fig. 2.13. *18th gestational week.* Hypoplasia of left fibula in VACTERL association. Small left foot with only one ray. Fused vertebrae L3–5 Segmentation errors and hypoplasia of the sacrum (caudal regression). Urethral pathology is suggested by narrow and asymmetric pubic bones. Other findings: esophageal atresia Vogt IIIb; anal atresia; absent urethra, bladder, and kidneys

Diagnosis	Accessory radiological findings in the fetus
Acrofacial dysostosis, type Rodriguez [1] MIM 201170	Phocomelia of arms, defective ulnar ray, short humerus, hypoplastic scapula
Camptomelic dysplasia; see p. 114	Bowing of femur and tibia, pear-shaped iliae; hypoplasia of claviculae, scapulae; cervical kyphosis
Chondroectodermal dysplasia Ellis van-Creveld [2]; see p. 137	Postaxial polydactyly; narrow chest; short, thick, bowed humeri and femurs; hypoplasia/aplasia tibiae; triradiate acetabula
Chromosome abnormalities	Rare
De la Chapelle dysplasia [3], including atelosteogenesis II; see p. 150 MIM 256050	Deficiency of fibular and ulnar rays; hemivertebrae; platyspondyly; coronal clefts; thin, short ribs
Du Pan brachydactyly, fibular aplasia [4]; see Grebe dysplasia p. 159 MIM 228900	Dislocation of elbow, knee, or hip; complex brachydactyly

Diagnosis	Accessory radiological findings in the fetus
Ectrodactyly-fibular aplasia [5] MIM 113310	Variable absence or hypoplasia of ulna, carpals, metacarpals, phalanges, fibulae, tarsals, metatarsals; brachydactyly; syndactyly; triphalangeal thumb
Femoral hypoplasia, unusual facies syndrome [6] MIM 134780	Small mandible, cleft palate, bowing of femur, hypoplastic/absent fibula or tibia, hypoplastic acetabula, preaxial polydactyly
Femur-fibula-ulna complex (FFU syndrome) [7]; see Fig. 2.14 MIM 228200	Asymmetric hypoplasia/aplasia of femur, fibula, humerus, ulna; humero-ulnar/radial synostosis; oligodactyly
Fibular aplasia/hypoplasia [8] Limb/pelvis-hypoplasia/aplasia syndrome [9] MIM 276820	Isolated defect of the fibula Hypoplastic femurs and feet; aplastic fibulae; oligodactyly; short, bent ulnae
Mesomelic dysplasias [10]; see p. 155	Different types and degrees of mesomelic shortening of the extremities with or without phalangeal involvement
Seckel syndrome [11] MIM 210600	Severe intrauterine growth retardation; microcephaly; craniosynostosis; absent fibula
VACTERL association; Fig. 2.13	Aplasia of fibula in rare cases (see: "Aplasia, Hypoplasia of Thumb and Radius")

References

1. Rodriguez JI, Palacios J, Urioste M (1992) Acrofacial dysostosis syndromes (letter). Am J Med Genet 42:851–852
2. Benjamin B, Omojola MF, Ashouri K (1991) Clinical and radiological features of chondroectodermal dysplasia. Ann Saudi Med 11:534–538
3. Sillence DO, Kozlowski K, Rogers JG et al (1987) Atelosteogenesis: evidence for heterogeneity. Pediatr Radiol 17:112–118
4. Langer LO Jr, Cervenka J, Camargo M (1989) A severe autosomal recessive acromesomelic dysplasia, the Hunter-Thompson type, and comparison with the Grebe type. Hum Genet 81:323–328
5. Rudiger RA, Haase W. Passarge E (1970) Association of ectrodactyly, ectodermal dysplasia, and cleft lip/palate. Am J Dis Child 120:160–163
6. Burn J, Winter RM, Baraitser M et al (1984) The femoral hypoplasia-unusual facies syndrome. J Med Genet 21:331–340
7. Lenz W, Zygulska M, Horst J (1993) FFU complex: an analysis of 491 cases. Hum Genet 91:347–356
8. Lewin SO, Opitz JM (1986) Fibular a/hypoplasia: review and documentation of the fibular developmental field. Am J Med Genet [Suppl] 2:215–238
9. Raas-Rothschild A, Goodman RM et al (1988) Pathological features and prenatal diagnosis in the newly-recognised limb/pelvis-hypoplasia/aplasia syndrome. J Med Genet 25:687–697
10. Kaitila II, Leisti T, Rimoin CL (1976) Mesomelic skeletal dysplasias. Clin Orthop 114:94–106
11. Majewski F, Goecke T (1982) Studies of microcephalic primordial dwarfism I: approach to a delineation of the Seckel syndrome. Am J Med Genet 12:7–21

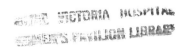

Femur: Aplasia, Hypoplasia

Aplasia or hypoplasia of the femur is rare, most often associated with other radiological signs helping to solve the differential diagnosis.

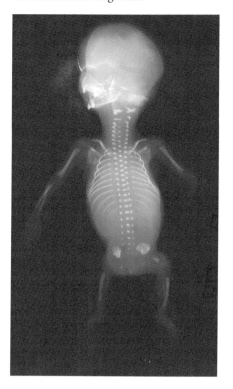

Fig. 2.14. *17th gestational week.* Complex tubular bone aplasia/hypoplasia in femur-fibula-ulna complex. Aplasia of the right femur, hypoplasia of the left femur, hypoplastic fibulae, aplasia of left radius, hypoplasia of the left ulna, two triphalangeal digits on the left

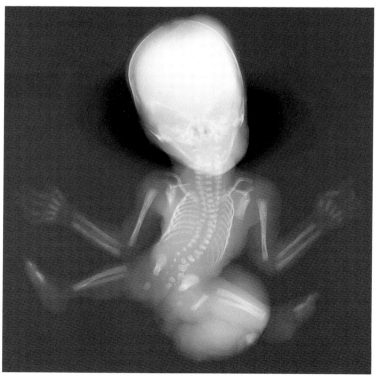

Fig. 2.15. *20th gestational week.* Femoral aplasia/hypoplasia in limb-body wall complex. Aplasia of the right femur, hypoplasia of left femur. Disproportionately short trunk. vertebral segmentation defects. Abdominal wall defect and bladder exstrophy. The upper extremities are normal

Diagnosis	Accessory radiological findings in the fetus
Diabetic embryopathy [1] see Fig. 2.36	Caudal regression, segmentation defects of the spine, defects of ulna and tibia
Ectrodactyly-tibial hypoplasia [2] MIM 119100	Split hand and/or foot, polydactyly, ulnar hypoplasia, tibial hypoplasia, bifid femur
Femoral hypoplasia, unusual facies syndrome [3] MIM 134780	Small jaw, cleft palate, radio-ulnar synostosis, absent fibula, absent tibia, hypoplastic acetabula, preaxial polydactyly of feet
Femur-fibula-ulna syndrome (FFU complex) [4]; Fig 2.14 MIM 228200	Asymmetric hypoplasia/aplasia of femur, fibula, humerus; humero-ulnar/-radial synostosis; oligodactyly
Limb, body wall complex [5]; Fig. 2.15 MIM 217100	Defect of lower abdominal wall, bladder exstrophy, pubic diastasis, segmental defects of lower extremities, spinal segmentation defects
Limb/pelvis-hypoplasia/aplasia syndrome [6] MIM 276820	Hypoplastic femur; aplasia of fibula; hypoplastic feet; oligodactyly; short, bent ulnae
Omodysplasia [7–9]; see p. 152 MIM 164745, 251455	Rhizomelia of upper limbs by distal hypoplasia of the humeri, milder involvement of lower limbs; dislocation of radial heads
Proximal focal femoral deficiency [10] MIM 228200	Unilateral short femur due to proximal reduction defect, hip joint preserved

References

1. Dunn V, Nixon GW, Jaffe RB, Condon VR (1981) Infants of diabetic mothers: radiographic manifestations. AJR 137:123–128
2. Majewski F, Kuster W, ter Haar B et al (1985) Aplasia of tibia with split-hand/split-foot deformity. Report of six families with 35 cases and considerations about variability and penetrance. Hum Genet 70:136–147
3. Burn J, Winter RM, Baraitser M et al (1984) The femoral hypoplasia-unusual facies syndrome. J Med Genet 21:331–340
4. Lenz W, Zygulska M, Horst J (1993) FFU complex: an analysis of 491 cases. Hum Genet 91:347–356
5. Higginbottom MC, Jones KL, Hall BD (1979) The amniotic band disruption complex: timing of amniotic rupture and variable spectra of consequent defects. J Pediatr 95:544–549
6. Raas-Rothschild A, Goodman RM et al (1988) Pathological features and prenatal diagnosis in the newly-recognised limb/pelvis-hypoplasia/aplasia syndrome. J Med Genet 25:687–697
7. Maroteaux P, Sauvegrain J, Chrispin A, Farriaux JP (1989) Omodysplasia. Am J Med Genet 32:371–375
8. Borochowitz Z, Barak M, Hershkowitz S (1991) Familial congenital micromelic dysplasia with dislocation of radius and distinct face: a new skeletal dysplasia syndrome. Am J Med Genet 39:91–96
9. Borochowitz Z, Barak M, Hershkowitz S (1995) Nosology of omodysplasia (letter). Am J Med Genet 58:377
10. Gillespie R, Torode IP (1983) Classification and management of congenital abnormalities of the femur. J Bone Joint Surg B 65:557–568

Femur: Bowing

Bowing of the femur is a quite common sign. It is helpful to evaluate at first whether length and structure are normal or not.

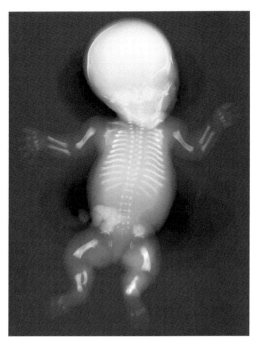

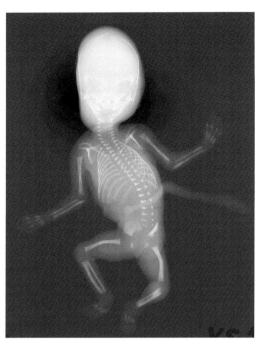

Fig. 2.16. *23rd gestational week.* Short bowed femora in thanatophoric dysplasia I. Narrow thorax, platyspondyly. All short and long tubular bones are markedly short and broad with flared and cupped metaphyses. Postaxial polydactyly right foot

Fig. 2.17. *15th gestational week.* Mild femoral bowing of the normally structured femora in Trisomy 18. Eleven pairs of ribs. Disharmonic skeletal maturation: absent ossification of the cervical vertebrae but well-ossified ischia

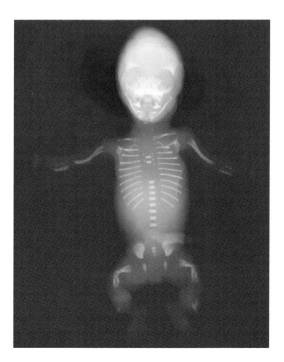

Fig. 2.18. *22nd gestational week.* Severe femoral bowing with deep metaphyseal defects in lethal hypophosphatasia. Erratic ossification of the vertebral bodies, absent ossification of the neural arches. Grossly defective, erratic ossification of the bones of the mesial and distal limb segments

Structure of femur	Diagnosis
A: short, normal structure; Fig. 2.16	Mostly lethal osteochondrodysplasias [4] (see Chap. 3, "Skeletal Dysplasias with Shortened Tubular Bones", p. 92 ff, "Skeletal Dysplasias with Congenital Bowing"), p. 110 ff; exception: kyphomelic dysplasia [1]
B: normal structure, slight bowing; Fig. 2.17	Unspecific radiological sign in many syndromes and chromosomal abnormalities with otherwise normal skeleton; exceptions: Antley-Bixler syndrome MIM 207410; campomelic dysplasia MIM 211970 (see p. 114)
C: abnormal structure, any size Osteogenesis imperfecta II [4], see p. 118 MIM 120150, MIM 166200 Hypophosphatasia, infantile form [2]; Fig. 2.18 MIM 241500 Neurofibromatosis I [5] MIM 162200	 Broad irregular diaphyses due to multiple fractures, multiple rib fractures, hypo-ossified calvarium Bowing of long bones, metaphyseal ossification defects, transverse midshaft spurs, hypo-ossified calvarium, erratic ossification of vertebrae Pseudarthrosis of femur (more often tibia)

References

1. Maclean RN, Prater WK, Lozzio CB (1983) Skeletal dysplasia with short, angulated femora (kyphomelic dysplasia). Am J Med Genet 14:373–380
2. Koslowski K, Sutcliffe J, Barylak A, Harrington G, Kemperdick H, Nolte K, Rheinwein H, Thomas PS, Unieck W (1976) Hypophosphatasia. Review of 24 cases. Pediatr Radiol 5;103–117
3. Fuhrmann W, Fuhrmann-Rieger A, de Sousa F (1980) Poly-, syn- and oligodactyly, aplasia or hypoplasia of fibula, hypoplasia of pelvis and bowing of femora in three sibs – a new autosomal recessive syndrome. Eur J Pediatr 133:123–129
4. Spranger J, Maroteaux P (1990) The lethal chondrodysplasias. Adv Hum Genet 19:1–103
5. Boero S, Catagni M, Donzelli O, Facchini R, Frediani PV (1997) Congenital pseudarthrosis of the tibia associated with neurofibromatosis-1: treatment with Illizarov's device. J Pediatr Orthop 17:675–685

Stippled Epiphyses – Stippled Ossification of Cartilage

For skeletal dysplasias with punctate calcifications see p. 138 ff (Greenberg dysplasia; dappled diaphysis dysplasia; chondrodysplasia punctata, different types; CHILD syndrome)

Definition:
– Syndromatic or symptomatic premature stippled calcification of epiphyses or apophyses of high radiographic density

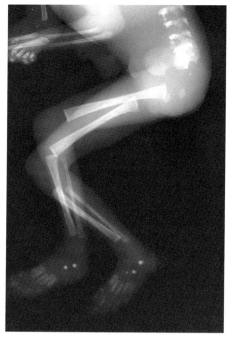

Fig. 2.19. *22nd gestational week.* Short femora in triploidy: femur length of 18th gestational week. Puncta in the tarsus and intervertebral disks

Diagnosis	Accessory radiological findings in the fetus
Chromosome abnormalities: Triploidy Trisomy 13 Trisomy 18 Trisomy 21 [1] Turner syndrome, X-Y translocation [2]	Besides the other signs which specific disorders expose (such as dystrophy, hypo-ossified calvaria, hypotelorism, nuchal cystic hygroma, umbilical hernia, radius aplasia, coronal vertebral clefts) most often only the calcaneus with a premature, dot-like, very dense ossification; especially in triploidy, intervertebral disks with a central calcification (see Fig. 2.19)
Fetal alcohol syndrome [3]	Intrauterine growth retardation, microcephaly, hemivertebra, Klippel-Feil syndrome
Hydantoin embryopathy [4] MIM 261720	Microcephaly, distal hyperphalangism or hypoplasia
Smith-Lemli-Opitz syndrome [5] MIM 270400	Growth retardation, microcephaly, postaxial polydactyly, split hand, clubfoot
Warfarin embryopathy [6, 7]	Short, broad hand; calcification of larynx and trachea; shortened limbs; occipital encephalocele
Zellweger syndrome [8] (cerebro-hepato-renal syndrome) MIM 214100	Microcephaly, no specific radiologic signs, stippled calcifications of the patella and mostly grouped around the pelvis

Chromosome 16p duplication, Zellweger Syndrome, DeBarsy-Syndrome (progeroid syndrome), show, except for stippled epiphyses, no other radiologic signs in the fetus helping to solve the differential diagnosis.

Single cases of undetermined origin have been published.

References

1. Sénécal J, Boguais MT, Le Berre C, Le Marec B (1968) Association d'une maladie des épiphyses ponctuees et d'une trisomie 21 chez un nouveau-né. Association of stippled epiphyses and trisomy 21 in a newborn infant. Arch Fr Pediatr 25:958–959
2. Morrison SC (1999) Punctate epiphyses associated with Turner syndrome. Pediatr Radiol 29:478–480
3. Leicher-Düber A, Schumacher R, Spranger J (1990) Stippled epiphyses in fetal alcohol syndrome. Pediatr Radiol 20:369–370
4. Wood BP, Young LM (1979) Pseudohyperphalangism in fetal Dilantin syndrome. Radiology 131:371–372
5. Dallaire L, Fraser FC (1969) The Smith-Lemli-Opitz syndrome of retardation, urogenital and skeletal anomalies. BDOAS 5:180–182
6. Happle R, Koch H, Lenz W (1980) The CHILD syndrome: congenital hemidysplasia with ichthyosiform erythroderma and limb defects. Eur J Pediatr 134:27–33
7. Tamburrini O, Iuri ABD, Guglielmo GLD (1987) Chondrodysplasia punctata after warfarin: case report with 18-month follow-up. Pediatr Radiol 17:323–324
8. Poznanski AK (1994) Punctate epiphyses: a radiological sign not a disease. Pediatr Radiol 24:418–424

Absent Hands/Feet

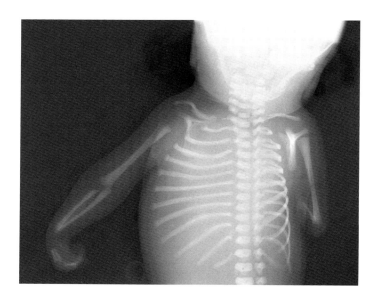

Fig. 2.20. *30th gestational week.* Complex aplasia/hypoplasia: aplasia of the left radius and hand in oromandibular-limb hypogenesis syndrome, hypoplasia of the left ulna. On the right side, slightly dysplastic radius and ulna, absent ossification of the 4th and 5th digits and of the phalanges of the 3rd digit

Diagnosis	Accessory radiological findings in the fetus
Acheiropodia [1] MIM 200500	Transverse terminal limb reductions, usually involving all extremities with variable deficiency of radius, ulna, humerus, tibia, and fibula; variable presence of Bohomoletz bone (hypoplastic bone at the tip of the upper limb stump with triphalangeal component)
Amniotic band disruption sequence [2] ADAM complex (Amniotic Deformity, Adhesions, Mutilations) MIM 217100	Usually asymmetric transverse terminal limb reductions/amputations and variable terminal syndactyly/pseudosyndactyly; may also include oligodactyly, hypoplasia of long bones, craniofacial and ventral wall disruption
Brachmann-de Lange syndrome [3, 4] MIM 122470 see Fig. 2.11, Fig. 2.21	Asymmetric and variable upper limb deficiency including absent or hypoplastic humerus, radius or ulna, carpals, metacarpals, and phalanges; other skeletal findings including microcephaly, micrognathia, supernumerary ribs, fused ribs, hemivertebrae, or vertebral fusion
Femur-fibula-ulna complex [5] MIM 228200	Asymmetric hypoplasia/aplasia of femur, fibula, ulna, humerus; humero-ulnar/-radial synostosis; oligodactyly
Holoprosencephaly-transverse limb defect [6]	Quadrilateral transverse terminal limb defects, holoprosencephaly
Oromandibular–limb hypogenesis syndromes; Fig. 2.20 Aglossia-adactylia Hypoglossia-hypodactylia Hanhart syndrome [7, 8] MIM 103300	Asymmetric and variable absent or hypoplastic humerus, radius, ulna, carpals, metacarpals, femur, tibia, fibula, tarsals, metatarsals; oligodactyly; syndactyly; microretrognathia; aplasia/hypoplasia of the tongue

References

1. Freire-Maia A, Laredo-Filho J, Freire-Maia N (1978) Genetics of acheiropodia ("The handless and footless families of Brazil"): X. Roentgenologic study. Am J Med Genet 2:321–330
2. Jones KL, Smith DW, Hall BW et al (1974) A pattern of craniofacial and limb defects secondary to aberrant tissue bands. J Pediatr 84:90–95
3. Pashayan HM, Fraser FC, Pruzansky S (1975) Variable limb malformations in the Brachmann-Cornelia de Lange syndrome. Birth Defects Orig Artic Ser 11:147–156
4. Kurlander FJ, DeMyer W (1967) Roentgenology of the Brachmann-de Lange syndrome. Radiology 88:101–110
5. Lenz W, Zygulska M, Horst J (1993) FFU complex: an analysis of 491 cases. Hum Genet 91:347–356
6. Slavotinek A, Stahlschmidt J, Moore L (1997) Transverse limb defects, holoprosencephaly and neuronal heterotopia – a new syndrome? Clin Dysmorphol 6:365–370
7. Hall BD (1971) Aglossia-adactylia. Birth Defects Orig Artic Ser 7:233–236
8. Kelln EE, Bennet CG, Klingberg WG (1968) Aglossia-adactylia syndrome. Am J Dis Child 116:549–552

Split/Cleft/Ectrodactyly of Hands and/or Feet

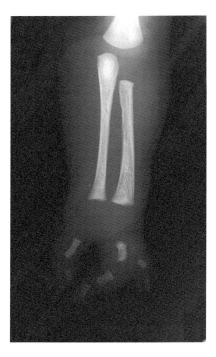

Fig. 2.21. *32nd gestational week.* Split hands with three incomplete rays bilaterally in Brachmann-de Lange syndrome

Diagnosis	Accessory radiological findings in the fetus
Acro-renal-mandibular syndrome [1] MIM 200980	Severe mandibular hypoplasia; variable and asymmetric limb reduction defects including hypoplastic or absent radius or tibia, oligodactyly, syndactyly, vertebral segmentation defects; other defects including renal agenesis/renal dysplasia, diaphragmatic hernia
Brachmann-de Lange syndrome [2]; Fig. 2.21 MIM 122470	Asymmetric and variable upper limb deficiency including absent or hypoplastic humerus, radius or ulna, carpals, metacarpals, and phalanges; other skeletal findings including microcephaly, micrognathia, supernumerary ribs, fused ribs; hemivertebrae or vertebral fusion
Chromosome abnormality trisomy 13 [3]	Microcephaly, hypotelorism, small orbits, hypo-ossification of calvarium, spinal dysraphism, hemivertebrae, absent/supernumerary/fused ribs, hypoplasia of pelvis, oligodactyly, polydactyly, syndactyly, camptodactyly, vertical talus; other defects including cardiac anomalies, omphalocele, holoprosencephaly, neural tube defect, cystic hygroma, hydrops fetalis

Diagnosis	Accessory radiological findings in the fetus
Chromosome abnormality trisomy 18 [4–7]	Microcephaly, hypo-ossification of calvarium, hypoplasia of maxilla and/or mandible, microretrognathia, absent or thin ribs, short sternum, spinal dysraphism, hypoplasia of pelvis, hypoplasia of first metacarpal, flexion deformities and overlapping fingers, vertical talus, short first toe, hammertoes; other defects: intrauterine growth retardation, cardiac anomalies, omphalocele, neural tube defect
DK phocomelia [8, 9] Phocomelia-encephalocele-thrombocytopenia-urogenital malformation von Voss-Cherstvoy syndrome MIM 223340	Microcephaly; encephalocele; absent or hypoplastic humerus, radius, ulna, metacarpals, thumbs; oligodactyly; syndactyly
Ectrodactyly-Ectodermal dysplasia – Clefting syndrome [10] MIM 129900	Cleft lip ± palate; variable absence or hypoplasia of carpals, metacarpals, tarsals, metatarsals, phalanges; variable oligodactyly; variable syndactyly; other finding: renal dysplasia
Ectrodactyly-fibular aplasia [11] MIM 113310	Variable absence or hypoplasia of ulna, carpals, metacarpals, phalanges, fibulae, tarsals, metatarsals; brachydactyly; syndactyly; triphalangeal thumb
Ectrodactyly, isolated malformation MIM 183600, MIM 313350, MIM 600095, MIM 605289, MIM 606708	Variable and usually asymmetric absence or hypoplasia of phalanges, metacarpals and/or metatarsals, carpals and/or tarsals, radius, ulna, tibia, and fibula
Ectrodactyly-tibial aplasia [12, 13] MIM 119100	Variable absence or hypoplasia of radius, ulna, carpals, metacarpals, phalanges, tibia, tarsals, metatarsals; bifid distal femur; bowed tibia, absent or hypoplastic patella; preaxial or postaxial polydactyly; variable oligodactyly; variable syndactyly; may present as four-extremity monodactyly or transverse hemimelia
Femur-fibula-ulna complex [13] MIM 228200	Asymmetric hypoplasia/aplasia of femur, fibula, ulna, humerus; humero-ulnar/radial synostosis; oligodactyly
Holoprosencephaly-hypertelorism-ectrodactyly syndrome [14]	Craniosynostosis, hypertelorism, absent or hypoplastic radius, ulna, phalanges; other defects: cleft lip ± palate, holoprosencephaly, neural tube defect
Monodactylous ectrodactyly and bifid femur Wolfgang-Gollop syndrome [15, 16] MIM 228250	Variable absence or hypoplasia of radius, ulna, carpals, metacarpals, phalanges, tibia, patella, tarsals, and metatarsals; bifid femur; talipes equinovarus; vertebral body fusion; hemivertebrae
Oromandibular–limb hypogenesis syndromes: aglossia-adactylia, hypoglossia-hypodactylia, Hanhart syndrome [17, 18]; see Fig. 2.4 MIM 103300	Asymmetric and variably absent or hypoplastic humerus, radius, ulna, carpals, metacarpals, femur, tibia, fibula, tarsals, and metatarsals; oligodactyly; syndactyly; microretrognathia

References

1. Halal F, Desgranges M-F, Leduc B et al (1980) Acro-renal–mandibular syndrome. Am J Med Genet 5:277–284

2. Braddock SR, Lachman RS, Stoppenhaggen CC et al (1993) Radiologic features in Brachmann-de Lange syndrome. Am J Med Genet 47:1006–1013

3. Urioste M, Martinez-Frias ML, Aparicio P (1994) Ectrodactyly in Trisomy 13 syndrome. Am J Med Genet 53:390–392

4. James AE Jr, Merz T, Janower ML et al (1971) Radiological features of the most common autosomal disorders: trisomy 21–22 (mongolism or Down's syndrome), trisomy 18, trisomy 13–15, and the cri du chat syndrome. Clin Radiol 22:417–433

5. Franceschini P, Fabris C, Ponzone A et al (1974) Skeletal alterations in Edwards' disease (trisomy 18 syndrome). Ann Radiol (Paris) 17:361–367

6. Rogers RC (1994) Trisomy 18 with unilateral atypical ectrodactyly. Am J Med Genet 49:125

7. Kjaer I, Keeling JW, Hansen BF (1996) Pattern of malformations in the axial skeleton in human trisomy 18 fetuses. Am J Med Genet 65:332–336

8. Cherstvoy E, Lazjuk G, Lurie I et al (1980) Syndrome of multiple congenital malformations including phocomelia, thrombocytopenia, encephalocele, and urogenital abnormalities Lancet 2:485

9. Lubinsky MS, Kahler SG, Speer IE et al (1994) von Voss-Cherstvoy syndrome: a variable perinatally lethal syndrome of multiple congenital anomalies. Am J Med Gent 52:272–278

10. Rudiger RA, Haase W, Passarge E (1970) Association of ectrodactyly, ectodermal dysplasia, and cleft lip/palate. Am J Dis Child 120:160–163

11. Evans JA, Reed MH, Greenberg CR (2002) Fibular aplasia with ectrodactyly. Am J Med Genet 113:52–58

12. Majewski F, Kuster W, ter Haar B et al (1985) Aplasia of tibia with split-hand/split-foot deformity. Report of six families with 35 cases and considerations about variability and penetrance. Hum Genet 70:136–147

13. Lenz W, Zygulska M, Horst J (1993) FFU complex: an analysis of 491 cases. Hum Genet 91:347–356

14. Hartsfield JK Jr, Bixler D, Demyer WE (1984) Syndrome identification case report 119: hypertelorism associated with holoprosencephaly and ectrodactyly. J Clin Dysmorph 2:27–31

15. Gollop TR, Lucchesi E, Martins RMM (1980) Familial occurrence of bifid femur and monodactylous ectrodactyly. Am J Med Genet 7:319–322

16. Raas-Rothschild A, Nir A, Ziv JB, Rein AJJT (1999) Agenesis of tibia with ectrodactyly/Gollop-Wolfgang complex associated with congenital heart malformations and additional skeletal abnormalities. Am J Med Genet 84:361–364

17. Hall BD (1971) Aglossia-adactylia. Birth Defects Orig Artic Ser 7:233–236

18. Kelln EE, Bennet CG, Klingberg WG (1968) Aglossia-adactylia syndrome. Am J Dis Child 116:549–552

Readers' Notes:

Preaxial Polydactyly of Hands and/or Feet

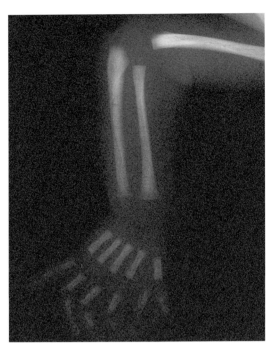

Fig. 2.22. *24th gestational week.* Preaxial polydactyly in Townes-Brock syndrome. Duplication of triphalangeal thumbs; defective ossification of the middle and distal phalanges. Other findings: imperforate anus, triphalangeal thumbs, ear anomalies

Diagnosis	Accessory radiological findings in the fetus
Aase syndrome [1] MIM 205600 Blackfan-Diamond syndrome Anemia and triphalangeal thumbs [2]	Broad thumb, triphalangeal thumb, hypoplastic thumb, radial hypoplasia, abnormal clavicles; other features: cleft palate, congenital heart defect, congenital hypoplastic anemia
Acrocallosal syndrome [3, 4] MIM200990	Macrocephaly, prominent forehead, large fontanelles, hypertelorism, bifid terminal phalanges of thumbs, duplicated hallux, syndactyly, brachydactyly, postaxial polydactyly; other features: absent corpus callosum, other brain defects, cleft palate, heart defect
Carpenter syndrome [5, 6] Acrocephalopolysyndactyly, type 2 MIM 201000	Craniosynostosis, Kleeblattschädel (cloverleaf skull), absence or hypoplasia of middle phalanges, double ossification center of proximal phalanx of thumb, postaxial polydactyly, broad first metatarsal, syndactyly, coxa valga, genu vara, pes varus
Chromosome abnormalities	Variable according to specific segmental aneuploidy
Diabetic embryopathy [7]	Hemivertebrae, absent or hypoplastic femora, hypoplastic tibia, postaxial polydactyly, spinal dysraphism, neural tube defect, congenital heart defect

Diagnosis	Accessory radiological findings in the fetus
Greig cephalopolysyndactyly [8, 9] MIM 175700	Macrocephaly, prominent forehead, large fontanelles, hypertelorism, postaxial polydactyly of hands (rarely of feet), broad thumbs, broad hallux
Holt-Oram syndrome [10, 11] Cardiomelic syndrome MIM 142900	Absent or hypoplastic humerus, radius, ulna, first metacarpal, and thumb; triphalangeal thumb; absent or hypoplastic carpals; delayed ossification or fusion of carpals; other polydactyly; radioulnar synostosis; hypoplasia of the clavicle and scapula; Sprengel anomaly; pectus excavatum or carinatum; rib hypoplasia or fusion; vertebral fusion or hemivertebra and scoliosis; other anomalies: cardiac defects (secundum type atrial septal defect the most common)
Hydrolethalus syndrome [13] MIM 236680	Macrocephaly, keyhole-shaped deformity of foramen magnum, severe micrognathia, postaxial polydactyly of hands, tibial hypoplasia, bowing of tubular long bones, duplicated hallux, hallux varus, short first metatarsal; other anomalies: major brain defects including hydrocephalus, cleft lip/palate, laryngotracheobronchial malformation, pulmonary hypoplasia
Isolated defect MIM 174400, 174500, 174700	May include postaxial polydactyly and syndactyly
Orofacial digital syndromes [14] Type I MIM 311200 Type II MIM 252100 Type IV MIM 258860 Type VI MIM 277170 Type VIII MIM 311200	Absence or hypoplasia of phalanges, metacarpals, metatarsals; clinodactyly; camptodactyly; forked or bifid metacarpals; duplication of hallux; postaxial polydactyly; irregular modeling of bones in hands and feet; syndactyly; tibial hypoplasia; talipes equinovarus; other features: microcephaly, lobulated or cleft tongue, cleft lip/palate, malformations of brain and other organs
Pfeiffer syndrome [15, 16] Acrocephalopolysyndactyly, type 5 MIM 101600	Craniosynostosis, Kleeblattschädel, hypertelorism, ocular proptosis/shallow orbits, broad first metacarpals and phalanges of the thumb, radial deviation of thumb, syndactyly, broad first metatarsals and phalanges of hallux, deviation of hallux, absence or hypoplasia of other phalanges, symphalangism, radioulnar or radiohumeral synostosis
Pseudo-trisomy 13 syndrome [17] MIM 264480	Microcephaly, micrognathia, hemivertebrae, absent or hypoplastic radius or ulna, postaxial polydactyly, absent or hypoplastic tibia, broad hallux, talipes equinovarus; other defects: omphalocele, malformations of brain and other organs
Short rib-polydactyly syndromes [18, 19], different types; see p. 133 MIM 269860, 263520	In common: short horizontal ribs, short tubular bones, postaxial polydactyly, hypoplastic ilia
Townes-Brocks syndrome [20, 21]; Fig. 2.22 MIM 107480	Bifid or broad thumb, triphalangeal thumb, syndactyly, clinodactyly, hypoplasia or absent carpals, carpal and/or tarsal fusion, pseudoepiphyses of metacarpals, metatarsal fusion other features: ear anomalies, imperforate anus

References

1. Aase JM, Smith DW (1969) Congenital anemia and triphalangeal thumbs: a new syndrome. J Pediatr 74:4171–4174
2. Alter BP (1978) Thumbs and anemia. Pediatrics 62:613–614
3. Schinzel A, Schmid W (1980) Hallux duplication, postaxial polydactyly, absence of the corpus callosum, severe mental retardation and additional anomalies in two unrelated patients: a new syndrome. Am J Med Genet 6:241–249
4. Gelman-Kohan Z, Antonelli J, Ankori-Cohen H et al (1991) Further delineation of the acrocallosal syndrome. Eur J Pediatr 150:797–799
5. Carpenter G (1901) Two sisters showing malformations of the skull and other congenital abnormalities. Rep Soc Study Dis Child 1:110–118
6. Cohen DM, Green JG, Miller J et al (1987) Acrocephalopolysyndactyly type II – Carpenter syndrome: clinical spectrum and an attempt at unification with Goodman and Summitt syndromes. Am J Med Gent 28:311–324
7. Becerra JE, Khoury MJ, Cordero JF et al (1990) Diabetes mellitus during pregnancy and the risks for specific birth defects: a population-based case-control study. Pediatrics 85:1–9
8. Greig DM (1926) Oxycephaly. Edinb Med J 33:189–218
9. Debeer P, Peeters H, Driess S et al (2003) Variable phenotype in Greig cephalopolysyndactyly syndrome: clinical and radiological findings in 4 independent families and 3 sporadic cases with identified GLI3 mutations. Am J Med Genet 120A:49–58
10. Holt M, Oram S (1960) Familial heart disease with skeletal malformations. Br Heart J 22:236–242
11. Poznanski AK, Gall JC Jr, Stern AM (1970) Skeletal manifestations of the Holt-Oram syndrome. Radiology 94:45–53
12. Salonen R, Herva R, Norio R (1981) The hydrolethalus syndrome; delineation of a "new" lethal malformation syndrome based on 28 patients. Clin Genet 19:321–330
13. Herva R, Seppanen U (1984) Roentgenologic findings of the hydrolethalus syndrome. Pediatr Radiol 14:41–43
14. Toriello HV (1993) Oral-facial-digital syndromes. Clin Dysmorph 2:95–105
15. Pfeiffer RA (1964) Dominant erbliche Akrocephalosyndaktylie. Z Kinderheilkd 90:301–320
16. Cohen MM Jr (1993) Pfeiffer syndrome update, clinical subtypes, and guidelines for differential diagnosis. Am J Med Genet 45:300–307
17. Cohen MM Jr, Gorlin RJ (1991) Pseudo-trisomy 13 syndrome. Am J Med Genet 39:332–335
18. Beemer FA, Langer LO Jr, Klep-de Pater JM et al (1983) A new short rib syndrome: report of two cases. Am J Med Genet 14:115–123
19. Spranger JW, Grimm B, Weller M et al (1974) Short rib-polydactyly (SRP) syndromes, types Majewski and Saldino-Noonan. Z Kinderheilkd 116:73–94
20. Townes PL, Brocks ER (1972) Hereditary syndrome of imperforate anus with hand, foot and ear anomalies. J Pediatr 81:321–326
21. Powell CM, Michaelis RC (1999) Townes-Brocks syndrome. J Med Genet 36:89–93

Readers' Notes:

Postaxial Polydactyly of Hands and/or Feet

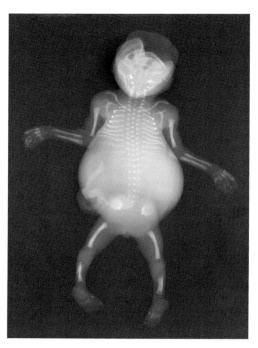

Fig. 2.23. *16th gestational week.* Postaxial polydactyly in Meckel-Gruber syndrome. Six toes, shortened tibia and fibula (mesomelia), slight bowing of femora. Ruptural encephalocele

Diagnosis	Accessory radiological findings in the fetus
Acrocallosal syndrome [1] MIM 200990	Macrocephaly, prominent forehead, large fontanelles, hypertelorism, bifid terminal phalanges of thumbs, duplicated hallux, preaxial polydactyly, syndactyly, brachydactyly: other features: absent corpus callosum, other brain defects, cleft palate, heart defect
Asphyxiating thoracic dystrophy [2, 3]; see p. 135 Jeune syndrome MIM 208500	Long narrow thorax with short, horizontal ribs, irregular costochondral junctions; short and flared iliac bones; triradiate acetabulae; ischial and pubic bones with medial and lateral spurs; premature ossification of the capital femoral epiphysis; shortened long tubular bones with irregular metaphyses; short and/or broad phalanges
Carpenter syndrome [4, 5] Acrocephalopolysyndactyly, type 2 MIM 201000	Craniosynostosis, Kleeblattschädel, absence or hypoplasia of middle phalanges, double ossification center of proximal phalanx of thumb, preaxial polydactyly, broad first metatarsal, syndactyly, coxa valga, genu vara, pes varus
Chromosome abnormality, trisomy 13 [6]	Microcephaly, hypotelorism, small orbits, hypo-ossification of calvarium, spinal dysraphism, hemivertebrae, absent/supernumerary/fused ribs, hypoplasia of pelvis, oligodactyly, syndactyly, camptodactyly, vertical talus: Other defects: heart defects, omphalocele, holoprosencephaly, neural tube defect, cystic hygroma, hydrops fetalis

Diagnosis	Accessory radiological findings in the fetus
Chromosome abnormality, other [6]	Variable according to specific segmental aneuploidy
Elejalde syndrome [7] Acrocephalopolydactylous dysplasia MIM 200995	Craniosynostosis, hypertelorism, shortening of all long bones: Other features: generalized overgrowth, cystic hygroma, hydrops fetalis, omphalocele
Ellis-van Creveld syndrome [8]; see p. 137 Chondroectodermal dysplasia MIM 225500	Mild narrowing of thorax with short ribs, small and flared ilia, triradiate acetabulae, short tubular long bones, bowing of humerus and femur, premature ossification of capital femoral epiphysis, hypoplasia of proximal tibial ossification center, genu valgum, short fibula, carpal fusion, short and broad middle phalanges, hypoplasia of distal phalanges, cone-shaped epiphyses of phalanges; other features: heart defect, sparse hair, hypoplastic nails, oral frenula
Focal dermal hypoplasia [9, 10] Goltz syndrome MIM 305600	Absent or hypoplastic clavicles; clavicular pseudoarthrosis; bifid or fused ribs; asymmetric oligodactyly; ectrodactyly; syndactyly; preaxial polydactyly; bifid thumb; bifid hallux; hemimelia; short phalanges, metacarpals, metatarsals; osteopathia striata; other features: skin, eye, and visceral malformations
Grebe syndrome [11, 12]; see p. 159 MIM 200700	Absent or hypoplastic proximal and middle phalanges; syndactyly; absent or hypoplastic metacarpals and carpals; carpal fusion; very short tubular long bones (lower limbs more severe than upper limbs); dislocated radial heads; aplasia/hypoplasia of ulna, radius, and femur
Greig cephalopolysyndactyly [13, 14] MIM 175700	Macrocephaly, prominent forehead, large fontanelles, hypertelorism, preaxial polydactyly of feet, broad thumbs, broad hallux
Hydrolethalus syndrome [15, 16] MIM 236680	Macrocephaly, keyhole-shaped deformity of foramen magnum, severe micrognathia, preaxial polydactyly, tibial hypoplasia, bowing of tubular long bones, duplicated hallux, hallux varus, short first metatarsal; other anomalies; major brain defects including hydrocephalus, cleft lip/palate, laryngotracheobronchial malformation, pulmonary hypoplasia
Isolated defect MIM 174200	May include preaxial polydactyly, syndactyly
Meckel-Gruber syndrome [17, 18]; Fig. 2.23 MIM 249000	Rarely preaxial polydactyly or bifid thumb, talipes equinovarus; other features: polycystic kidneys; CNS anomalies including microcephaly, occipital encephalocele (most common), Dandy-Walker malformation, hydrocephalus
Orofacial digital syndromes [19] Type II MIM 252100 Type III MIM 258850 Type IV MIM 252100 Type V MIM 174300 Type VI MIM 277170 Type VIII MIM 311200	Absent or hypoplastic of phalanges, metacarpals, metatarsals; clinodactyly; camptodactyly, forked or bifid metacarpals; duplication of hallux; preaxial polydactyly; irregular modeling of bones in hands and feet; syndactyly; tibial hypoplasia; talipes equinovarus; other features: microcephaly, lobulated or cleft tongue, cleft lip/palate, malformations of brain and other organs

Diagnosis	Accessory radiological findings in the fetus
Pallister-Hall syndrome [20] MIM 146510	Central polydactyly, bifid third metacarpal, hypoplastic fourth metacarpal, metacarpal synostosis, syndactyly, subluxation or dislocation of radial head, mild shortening of long tubular bones, bifid hallux;. other features: hypothalamic hamartoma, imperforate anus, laryngeal cleft, visceral defects
Pseudo-trisomy 13 syndrome [21] MIM 264480	Microcephaly, micrognathia, hemivertebrae, absent or hypoplastic radius or ulna, preaxial polydactyly, absent or hypoplastic tibia, broad hallux, talipes equinovarus; Other defects: include omphalocele, malformations of brain and other organs
Short rib-polydactyly syndromes, different types [22–26]; see p. 133 ff MIM 263530, 263510, 263520, 269860	In common: relative macrocephaly, very short horizontal ribs, short tubular long bones, hypoplasia of scapula, small ilia, preaxial polydactyly
Simpson-Golabi-Behmel syndrome [27] MIM 312870	Macrocephaly, supernumerary ribs, vertebral anomalies, hypoplasia of distal phalanges, syndactyly, clinodactyly, broad hallux other features: hepatosplenomegaly, congenital heart defect, diaphragmatic hernia, renal dysplasia, and hydrops fetalis
Smith-Lemli-Opitz syndrome [28, 29] Type I MIM 270400 Type II MIM 268670	Microcephaly, micrognathia, thin ribs, hypoplastic first metacarpal, brachydactyly, syndactyly, talipes equinovarus, vertical talus; other features include CNS anomalies, cleft palate, heart defect, renal dysplasia, hydrops fetalis, genital hypoplasia, sex reversal

References

1. Schinzel A, Schmid W (1980) Hallux duplication, postaxial polydactyly, absence of the corpus callosum, severe mental retardation and additional anomalies in two unrelated patients: a new syndrome. Am J Med Genet 6:241–249
2. Langer LO Jr (1968) Thoracic-pelvic-phalangeal dystrophy: asphyxiating thoracic dystrophy of the newborn, infantile thoracic dystrophy. Radiology 91:447–456
3. Oberklaid F, Danks DM, Mayne V et al (1977) Asphyxiating thoracic dysplasia: clinical radiological and pathological information on 10 patients. Arch Dis Child 52:758–765
4. Carpenter G (1901) Two sisters showing malformations of the skull and other congenital abnormalities. Rep Soc Study Dis Child 1:110–118
5. Cohen DM, Green JG, Miller J et al (1987) Acrocephalopolysyndactyly type II – Carpenter syndrome: clinical spectrum and an attempt at unification with Goodman and Summitt syndromes. Am J Med Gent 28:311–324
6. James AE Jr, Merz T, Janower ML et al (1971) Radiological features of the most common autosomal disorders: trisomy 21–22 (mongolism or Down's syndrome), trisomy 18, trisomy 13–15, and the cri du chat syndrome. Clin Radiol 22:417–433
7. Elejalde BR, Giraldo C, Jimenez R et al (1977) Acrocephalopolydactylous dysplasia. Birth Defects Orig Artic Ser 13:53–67
8. Ellis RWB, van Creveld S (1940) A syndrome characterized by ectodermal dysplasia, polydactyly, chondro-dysplasia and congenital morbus cordis: report of three cases. Arch Dis Child 15:65–84
9. Goltz RW, Henderson RR, Hitch JM et al (1970) Focal dermal hypoplasia syndrome: a review of the literature and report of two cases. Arch Derm 101:1–11
10. Boothroyd AE, Hall CM (1988) The radiological features of Goltz syndrome: focal dermal hypoplasia. A report of two cases. Skeletal Radiol 17:505–508
11. Grebe H (1952) Die Achondrogenesis: ein einfach rezessives Erbmerkmal. Folia Hered Path 2:23–28
12. Costa T, Ramsby G, Cassia F et al (1998) Grebe syndrome: clinical and radiographic findings in affected individuals and heterozygous carriers. Am J Med Genet 75:523–529
13. Debeer P, Peeters H, Driess S et al (2003) Variable phenotype in Greig cephalopolysyndactyly syndrome: clinical and radiological findings in 4 independent families and 3 sporadic cases with identified GLI3 mutations. Am J Med Genet 120A:49–58
14. Greig DM (1926) Oxycephaly. Edinb Med J 33:189–218
15. Salonen R, Herva R, Norio R (1981) The hydrolethalus syndrome; delineation of a "new" lethal malformation syndrome based on 28 patients. Clin Genet 19:321–330
16. Herva R, Seppanen U (1984) Roentgenologic findings of the hydrolethalus syndrome. Pediatr Radiol 14:41–43
17. Kjaer KW, Fischer Hansen B, Keeling JW, Kjaer I (1999) Skeletal malformations in fetuses with Meckel syndrome. Am J Med Genet 84:469–475
18. Salonen R, Paavola P (1998) Meckel syndrome. J Med Genet 35:497–501

19. Toriello HV (1993) Oral-facial-digital syndromes. Clin Dysmorph 2:95–105

20. Hall JG, Pallister PD, Clarren SK (1980) Congenital hypothalamic hamartoblastoma, hypopituitarism, imperforate anus, and post-axial polydactyly– a new syndrome? Part I: clinical, causal, and pathogenetic considerations. Am J Med Genet 7:47–74

21. Cohen MM Jr, Gorlin RJ (1991) Pseudo-trisomy 13 syndrome. Am J Med Genet 39:332–335

22. Saldino RM, Noonan CD (1972) Severe thoracic dystrophy with striking micromelia, abnormal osseous development, including the spine, and multiple visceral anomalies. Am J Roentgenol 114:257–263

23. Verma IC, Bhargava S, Agarwal S (1975) An autosomal recessive form of lethal chondrodystrophy with severe thoracic narrowing, rhizoacromelic type of micromelia, polydactyly and genital anomalies. Birth Defects Orig Artic Ser 11:167–174

24. Naumoff P, Young LW, Mazer W et al (1977) Short-rib-polydactyly syndrome type 3. Radiology 122:443–447

25. Spranger JW, Grimm B, Weller M et al (1974) Short rib-polydactyly (SRP) syndromes, type Majewski and Saldino-Noonan. Z Kinderheilkd 116:73–94

26. Beemer FA, Langer LO Jr, Klep-de Pater JM et al (1983) A new short rib syndrome: report of two cases. Am J Med Genet 14:115–123

27. Chen E, Johnson JP, Cox VA et al (1993) Simpson-Golabi-Behmel syndrome: congenital diaphragmatic hernia and radiologic findings in two patients and follow-up of a previously reported case. Am J Med Genet 46:574–578

28. Smith DW, Lemli L, Opitz JM (1964) A newly recognized syndrome of multiple congenital anomalies. J Pediatr 64:210–217

29. Curry CJR, Carey JC, Holland JS et al (1987) Smith-Lemli-Opitz type II: multiple congenital anomalies with male pseudohermaphroditism and frequent early lethality. Am J Med Genet 26:45–57

Premature Cranial Synostosis/Cloverleaf Skull

Fibroblast growth factor receptor mutations cause some of the main short-limb skeletal dysplasias and craniosynostosis syndromes, of which some present a cloverleaf skull (Kleeblattschädel) [1].

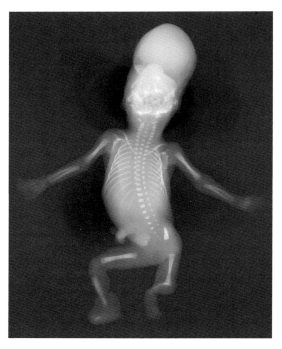

Fig. 2.24. *17th gestational week.* Cloverleaf skull in amnion band disruption sequence. Amputation of distal phalanges, aplasia of left tibia, ring constriction at the right shank with distal edema

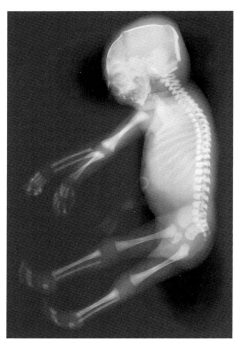

Fig. 2.25. *29th gestational week.* Premature craniosynostosis (donkey's back deformity of the coronal suture) in microcephalic Seckel syndrome with lissencephaly. Very thick calvaria

Diagnosis	Accessory radiological findings in the fetus
Acrocephalosyndactyly I (Apert) [1] Acrocephalosyndactyly V (Pfeiffer) [1] Acrocephalopolydactyly II (Carpenter) [1] MIM 101200, 101600, 201000	Distal bony syndactyly of hands and feet Occasionally duplication of first toe Preaxial poly-syndactyly of feet
Amniotic band disruption sequence ADAM complex (Amniotic Deformity, Adhesions and Mutilations) [2]; Fig. 2.24 Limb-body wall complex MIM 217100	Usually asymmetric transverse terminal limb reductions/amputations and variable terminal syndactyly/pseudosyndactyly; may also include oligodactyly, hypoplasia of long bones, craniofacial and ventral wall disruption
Antley-Bixler syndrome [3]; see p. 116 MIM 207410	Synostosis of coronal and lambdoid sutures, depression of nasal bridge, frontal bossing, radiohumeral synostosis, bowing of ulnae and femora, fractures
Baller-Gerold Syndrome [4] MIM 218600	Asymmetric radial defect; shortened bowed ulna; variable premature craniosynostosis (coronal suture most commonly)

Diagnosis	Accessory radiological findings in the fetus
Cloverleaf skull-limb anomalies, type Holtermüller-Wiedemann [5] MIM 148800	Trilobed skull deformity, ankylosis of the elbows
Craniosynostosis, nonsyndromic isolated	No further radiologic signs
M. Crouzon [6, 7] MIM 123500	Coronal and lambdoid suture synostosis, frontal bossing, midface hypoplasia, brachycephaly
Osteocraniostenosis [8, 9]; see p. 127	Intrauterine dwarfism, thin ribs, slender long bones with diaphyseal fractures, hypo-ossified calvaria, craniostenosis with mild cloverleaf skull appearance
Osteoglophonic dysplasia [10] MIM 166250	Bizarre premature cranial synostosis, rhizomelia, metaphyseal defects
Seckel syndrome [11]; Fig. 2.25 MIM 210600 Lissencephaly syndromes [12] MIM 247200	Severe intrauterine growth retardation, microcephaly, craniosynostosis, absent fibula
Short rib (polydactyly) syndrome Beemer-Langer type [13]; see p. 134 MIM 269860	Intrauterine dwarfism; short ribs; narrow thorax; marked bowing of long bones, especially radius and ulna; hydrops; pre-postaxial polydactyly
Thanatophoric dysplasia II [1]; see p. 94 MIM 187600	Short stature, short ribs, platyspondyly, mild shortening of long bones, straight femora

Such malformations can be also seen in some partial trisomy syndromes of chromosome 4, 9, 13.

References

1. Cohen MM (1997) Short-limb skeletal dysplasias and craniosynostosis: what do they have in common? Pediatr Radiol 27: 442–446
2. Jones KL, Smith DW, Hall BW et al (1974) A pattern of craniofacial and limb defects secondary to aberrant tissue bands. J Pediatr 84: 90–95
3. Hassell S, Butler MG (1994) Antley-Bixler syndrome: report of a patient and review of literature. Clin Genet 46: 372–376
4. Boudreaux JM, Colon MA, Lorusso GD et al (1990) Baller-Gerold syndrome: an 11th case of craniosynostosis and radial aplasia. Am J Med Genet 37: 447–450
5. Holtermüller K, Wiedemann H-R (1960) Kleeblattschädel-Syndrom. Med Monatsschr 14: 439–446
6. Kjaer I, Hansen BF, Kjaer KW, Skovby F (2000) Abnormal timing in the prenatal ossification of vertebral column and hand in Crouzon syndrome. Am J Med Genet 90: 386–389
7. Escobar LF, Bixler D, Padilla LM (1993) Quantitation of craniofacial anomalies in utero: fetal alcohol and Crouzon syndromes and thanatophoric dysplasia. Am J Med Genet 45: 25–29
8. Maroteaux P, Cohen-Solal L et al (1988) Lethal syndromes with thin bones (in French – summary in English). Arch Fr Pediatr 45: 477–481
9. Verloes A, Narcy F, Grattagliano B et al (1994) Osteocraniostenosis. J Med Genet 31: 772–778
10. Kelley RI, Borns PF, Nichols D, Zackai EH (1983) Osteoglophonic dwarfism in two generations. J Med Genet 20: 436–440
11. Majewski F, Goecke T (1982) Studies of microcephalic primordial dwarfism I: approach to a delineation of the Seckel syndrome. Am J Med Genet 12: 7–21
12. Aicardi J (1989) The lissencephaly syndromes. Int Pediatr 4: 118–126
13. Benallegue A, Lacete F, Maroteaux P (1987) Cloverleaf skull with generalised bone dysplasia close to asphyxiating thoracic dysplasia (in French – summary in English). Ann Genet (Paris) 30: 113–117

Unossified and Hypo-ossified Calvaria

Some skeletal dysplasias, such as atelosteogenesis, boomerang dysplasia, dappled diaphysis dysplasia, lethal male Melnick-Needles syndrome, and others, show a hypo-ossification of the calvaria. These all show striking additional skeletal findings (see p. 138, 148).

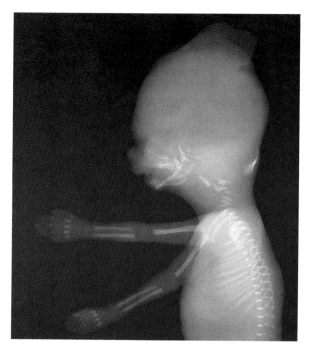

Fig. 2.26. *15th gestational week.* Unossified calvaria. in Trisomy 18

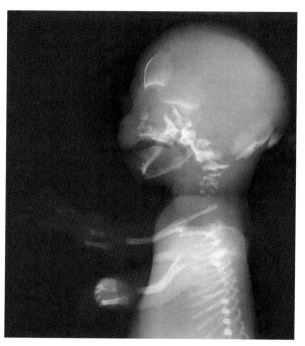

Fig. 2.27. *22nd gestational week.* Deficient calvarial ossification in lethal hypophosphatasia. Absent ossification of a major part of the spine. Incomplete or missing ossification of metacarpals and phalanges. Bowing of humeri with deep metaphyseal defects

Diagnosis	Accessory radiological findings in the fetus
Acalvaria [1]	May be associated with omphalocele, spina bifida
Aminopterin/methotrexate fetopathy [2] MIM 600325	Retardation, mesomelia of upper limbs
Angiontensin converting enzyme (ACE) inhibitor fetopathy [3]	Growth retardation, severely underossified calvarial bones
Chromosome abnormality [4]; Fig. 2.26, see Fig. 2.40 Trisomy 13 and 18	Intrauterine growth retardation microcephaly, hypo-ossification of calvarium, hypoplasia of maxilla and/or mandible, microretrognathia, absent or thin ribs, short sternum, spinal dysraphism
Hyperparathyroidism, neonatal familial [5] MMI 239200	Gross underossification, subperiosteal bone resorption, metaphyseal fractures (resembling mucolipidosis type II)

Diagnosis	Accessory radiological findings in the fetus
Hypophosphatasia, infantile form [6]; Fig. 2.27 MIM 241500	Poorly ossified skeleton, erratic ossification of vertebrae, deep metaphyseal defects, angulation of long bones, especially femur (see Femur: Bowing)
Osteocraniostenosis [7, 8]; see p. 127	Intrauterine dwarfism, thin ribs, slender long bones with diaphyseal fractures, hypo-ossified calvaria, craniostenosis with mild cloverleaf skull appearance
Osteogenesis imperfecta II [9]; see p. 118 MIM 120150, 166200	Multiple fractures of ribs and long bones, shortening and angulation of long bones. hypo-ossification present in all types

References

1. Harris CP, Townsend JJ, Carey JC (1993) Acalvaria: a unique congenital anomaly. Am J Med Genet 46:694–699
2. Brandner M, Nusslé D (1969) Foetopathie due à l'aminopterine avec sténose congénitale de l'espace médullaire des os tubularies longs. Ann Radiol (Paris) 12:703–710
3. Barr M Jr, Cohen MM Jr (1991) ACE inhibitor fetopathy and hypocalvaria: the kidney-skull connection. Teratology 44:485–495
4. Franceschini P, Fabris C, Ponzone A et al (1974) Skeletal alterations in Edwards' disease (trisomy 18 syndrome). Ann Radiol (Paris) 17:361–367
5. Eftekhari F, Yousefzadeh DK (1982) Primary infantile hyperparathyroidism: clinical, laboratory and radiographic features in 21 cases. Skeletal Radiol 8:201–208
6. Kozlowski K, Sutcliffe J, Barylak A, Harrington G, Kemperdick H, Nolte K, Rheinwein H, Thomas PS, Uniecka W (1976) Hypophosphatasia. Review of 24 cases. Pediatr Radiol 5:103–117
7. Kozlowski K, Kan A (1988) Intrauterine dwarfism, peculiar facies and thin bones with multiple fractures – a new syndrome. Pediatr Radiol 18:394–398
8. Verloes A, Narcy F, Grattagliano B et al (1994) Osteocraniostenosis. J Med Genet 31:772–778
9. Spranger J, Maroteaux P (1990) The lethal chondrodysplasias. Adv Hum Genet 19:1–103

Differential Diagnosis of Encephalocele

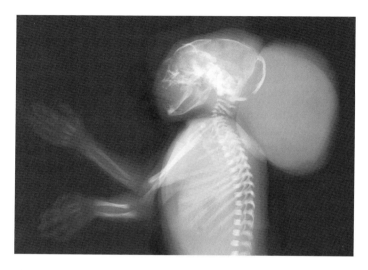

Fig. 2.28. *23rd gestational week.* Microcephaly with encephalocele. Note lückenschädel (craniolacunia)

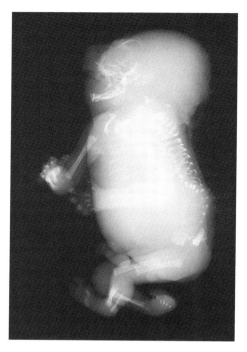

Fig. 2.29. *15th gestational week.* Iniencephaly. Retroflexion of head, "missing" neck by fusion of the soft tissue of the head and the shoulders. Defective ossification of the spine. Thoracolumbar kyphosis

Diagnosis	Accessory radiological findings in the fetus
Amniotic band disruption sequence [1] ADAM complex (*A*mniotic *D*eformity, *A*dhesions, *M*utilations) Limb-body wall complex MIM 217100	Usually asymmetric transverse terminal limb reductions/amputations and variable terminal syndactyly/pseudosyndactyly. May also include oligodactyly, hypoplasia of long bones, craniofacial and ventral wall disruption.
Chromosome abnormalities	Variable according to specific segmental aneuploidy
DK phocomelia [2] Phocomelia-encephalocele-thromobocytopenia-urogenital malformation von Voss-Cherstvoy syndrome MIM 223340	Microcephaly; absent or hypoplastic humerus, radius, ulna, metacarpals, thumb; oligodactyly; syndactyly of fingers; other features: genitourinary, cardiac anomalies, platelet abnormalities
Dyssegmental dysplasia; see p. 146 Silverman-Handmaker type [3, 4] MIM 224410	Severe irregularity in shape and size of vertebral bodies; hypoplastic thorax with short ribs; short and wide, bowed tubular long bones with wide metaphyses (dumbbell-shaped); hypoplasia of basilar portions of ilia; broad and thick ischium and pubis
Isolated finding; Fig. 2.28	Isolated encephalocele, microcephalus, no other radiologic findings.

Diagnosis	Accessory radiological findings in the fetus
Iniencephaly [5]; Fig. 2.29	Cervical spinal retroflexion, elevated face, occipito-spinal association, cervical spina bifida, rhizomelia of upper limbs, omphalocele
Meckel-Gruber syndrome [6]; see Fig. 2.23 MIM 249000	Post-axial polydactyly, rarely pre-axial polydactyly, talipes equinovarus; other features: polycystic kidneys; CNS anomalies including microcephaly, anencephaly, Dandy-Walker malformation, hydrocephalus
Roberts syndrome [7] Roberts-SC phocomelia syndrome Pseudothalidomide syndrome MIM 268300	Microcephaly, wormian bones, sometimes craniostenosis, hypertelorism, cleft lip and palate, variable absence or hypoplasia of tubular bones (usually asymmetric, and upper limbs typically more severe than lower limbs), fusion of tubular long bones, bowing of tubular long bones, contractures of large joints, absent carpals, absent first metacarpal and thumb, absent fifth metacarpal and phalanges, clinodactyly, syndactyly, talipes equinovarus or equinovalgus, calcaneovalgus: anomalies common in CNS, heart, kidneys
VACTERL association with hydrocephalus [8] MIM 276950	See "Aplasia, Hypoplasia of Thumb and Radius"
Walker-Warburg syndrome [9] Hydrocephalus, agyria, retinal dysplasia-encephalocele HARD ± E syndrome MIM 236670	Microcephaly, wide or delayed fusion of cranial sutures, joint contractures, talipes equinovarus; other features: retinal dysplasia, cataract, ear anomalies, Dandy-Walker malformation, hydrocephalus, heart defect
Warfarin embryopathy [10] Coumadin embryopathy Fetal warfarin syndrome	Frontal bossing; depressed nasal bridge; very small/short anteverted nose; short tubular long bones; short metacarpals, metatarsals, and phalanges; stippling or punctate calcification of epiphyses, spine, proximal femur, and calcaneus

References

1. Jones KL, Smith DW, Hall BW et al (1974) A pattern of craniofacial and limb defects secondary to aberrant tissue bands. J Pediatr 84:90–95
2. Cherstvoy E, Lazjuk G, Lurie I et al (1980) Syndrome of multiple congenital malformations including phocomelia, thrombocytopenia, encephalocele and urogenital abnormalities Lancet 2:485
3. Handmaker SD, Robinson LD, Campbell JA et al (1977) Dyssegmental dwarfism: a new syndrome of lethal dwarfism. Birth Defects Orig Art Ser 13:79–90
4. Spranger J, Maroteaux P (1990) The lethal chondrodysplasias. Adv Hum Genet 19:1–103
5. Lemire RJ, Beckwith JB, Shepard TH (1972) Iniencephaly and anencephaly with spinal retroflexion. A comparative study of eight human specimens. Teratology 6:27–36
6. Salonen R, Paavola P (1998) Meckel syndrome. J Med Genet 35:497–501
7. Freeman MV, Williams DW, Schimke RN et al (1974) The Roberts syndrome. Clin Genet 5:1–16
8. Vandenborne K, Beemer F, Fryns JP (1993) VACTERL with hydrocephalus. A distinct entity with a variable spectrum of multiple congenital anomalies. Genet Counsel 4:199–201
9. Pagon RA, Clarren SK, Milam DF et al (1983) Autosomal recessive eye and brain anomalies: Warburg syndrome. J Pediatr 102:542–546
10. Hall JG, Pauli RM, Wilson KM (1980) Maternal and fetal sequelae of anticoagulation during pregnancy. Am J Med Genet 68:122–140

Anencephaly/Myelomeningocele/Spina Bifida

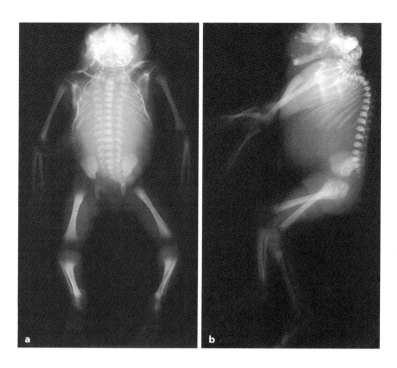

Fig. 2.30a, b. *29th gestational week.* Anencephaly with total craniorachischisis, aplasia of the cranial vault. Wide open spinal canal, severe kyphosis and swan's neck deformity of the cervical spine resulting in a disproportionately short trunk

Diagnosis	Accessory radiological findings in the fetus
Amniotic band disruption sequence ADAM complex (*A*mniotic *D*eformity, *A*dhesions, *M*utilations) Limb-body wall complex [1] MIM 217100	Usually asymmetric transverse terminal limb reductions/amputations and variable terminal syndactyly/pseudosyndactyly; may also include oligodactyly, hypoplasia of long bones, craniofacial and ventral wall disruption
CHILD syndrome [2] (*C*ongenital *h*emidysplasia, *i*chthyosiform erythroderma, *l*imb *d*efects) MIM 308050	Unilateral hypoplasia of limb(s) including absent or hypoplastic scapula, humerus, radius, ulna, femur, tibia, fibula; joint contracture or pterygium; punctate epiphyseal calcification; other features: congenital ichthyosiform erythroderma ipsilateral to limb deficiency, visceral anomalies
Chromosome abnormality trisomy 18 (Edward syndrome) [3]	Intrauterine growth retardation; microcephaly; prominent occiput; micrognathia; thin or absent ribs; short sternum; absent or hypoplastic radius, first metacarpal, thumb; camptodactyly; vertical talus; talipes equinovarus; short or dorsiflexed great toe; other defects: tracheoesophageal fistula, heart defect, absent or cystic kidneys, omphalocele
Chromosome abnormalities, other	Variable according to specific segmental aneuploidy
Diabetic embryopathy [4]	Hemivertebrae, absent or hypoplastic femora, hypoplastic tibia, preaxial or postaxial polydactyly, spinal dysraphism, neural tube defect, congenital heart defect

Diagnosis	Accessory radiological findings in the fetus
Fetal aminopterin syndrome Folate antagonist chemotherapeutic agents [5]	Delayed mineralization of calvarium, craniolacunae, craniosynostosis, hypertelorism, micrognathia, rib anomalies including fusion, joint contractures, absence or hypoplasia of digits including thumbs, syndactyly, talipes equinovarus
Fetal valproate syndrome [6, 7]	Prominent metopic ridge, bifrontal narrowing, clinodactyly, distal phalangeal hypoplasia, absent or hypoplastic radius, absent or hypoplastic thumb, talipes equinovarus
Isolated defect with or without rachischisis [8]; Fig. 2.30a, b	No other radiological signs
Laterality sequence [9] MIM 304570	Visceral heterotaxy, sacral agenesis.
Meckel-Gruber syndrome [10, 11]; see Fig. 2.23 MIM 249000	Post-axial polydactyly, rarely pre-axial polydactyly, talipes equinovarus;. other features include polycystic kidneys; CNS anomalies including microcephaly, occipital encephalocele (most common), Dandy-Walker malformation, hydrocephalus
Omphalocele-exstrophy of the bladder-imperforate anus-spinal defect (OEIS) complex [12] MIM 258040	Hemivertebrae, absent sacrum, widely spaced pubic bones, spinal dysraphism, talipes equinovarus, ventral wall defect
Pentalogy of Cantrell [13] Thoracoabdominal syndrome; see Fig. 2.39 MIM 313850	Sternal defects including agenesis, clefting or bifid sternum, absence of lower third of sternum; other defects include supraumbilical midline defect (omphalocele), central diaphragmatic hernia, pericardial defect, congenital heart defect
Short-rib polydactyly syndrome, type II (Majewski type) [14, 15]; see p. 136 MIM 263520	Relative macrocephaly, prominent forehead, thoracic hypoplasia with protuberant abdomen, short and horizontal ribs, short tubular long bones, ovoid tibia smaller than fibula, preaxial or postaxial polydactyly; other features include hydrops fetalis, cleft or lobulated tongue, multiple visceral and brain anomalies

References

1. Keeling JW, Kjaer I (1994) Diagnostic distinction between anencephaly and amnion rupture sequence based on skeletal analysis. J Med Gent 31:823–829
2. Happle R, Koch H, Lenz W (1980) The CHILD syndrome: congenital hemidysplasia with ichthyosiform erythroderma and limb defects. Eur J Pediatr 134:27–33
3. Nisani R, Chemke J, Cohen-Ankori H et al (1981) Neural tube defects in trisomy 18. Prenat Diag 1:227–231
4. Zacharias JF, Jenkins, JH, Marion JP (1984) The incidence of neural tube defects in the fetus and neonate of the insulin-dependent diabetic woman. Am J Obstet Gynecol 150:797–798
5. Milunsky A, Graef JW, Gaynor MJF (1968) Methotrexate induced congenital malformations with a review of the literature. J Pediatr 72:790–795
6. Robert E, Guibaud P (1982) Maternal valproic acid and congenital neural tube defects. Lancet 2:937
7. Sharony R, Garber A, Viskochil D et al (1993) Preaxial ray reduction defects as part of valproic acid embryofetopathy. Prenatal Diag 13:909–918
8. David T, Nixon A (1976) Congenital malformations associated with anencephaly and iniencephaly. J Med Genet 13:263–265

9. Casey B, Devoto M, Jones KL et al (1993) Mapping a gene for familial situs abnormalities to human chromosome Xq24–27.1. Nat Genet 5:403–407
10. Salonen R, Paavola P (1998) Meckel syndrome. J Med Genet 35:497–501
11. Seppanen U, Herva R (1983) Roentgenologic features of the Meckel syndrome. Pediatr Radiol 13:329–331
12. Carey JC, Greenbaum, B, Hall BD (1978) The OEIS Complex (omphalocele, exstrophy, imperforate anus, spinal defects). Birth Defects Orig Artic Ser 14:253–263
13. Hori A, Roessmann U, Eubel R et al (1984) Exencephaly in Cantrell-Haller-Ravitsch syndrome. Acta Neuropathol 65:158–162
14. Martinez-Frias ML, Bermejo E, Urioste M et al (1993) Short rib-polydactyly syndrome (SROS) with anencephaly and other central nervous system anomalies: a new type of SRPS or a more severe expression of a known SRPS entity? Am J Med Genet 47:782–787
15. Spranger JW, Grimm B, Weller M et al (1974) Short rib-polydactyly (SRP) syndromes, types Majewski and Saldino-Noonan. Z Kinderheilkd 116:73–94

Vertebral Segmentation Defects/Hemivertebrae/Vertebral Fusion

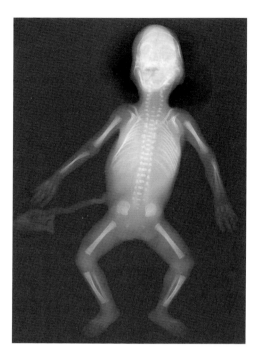

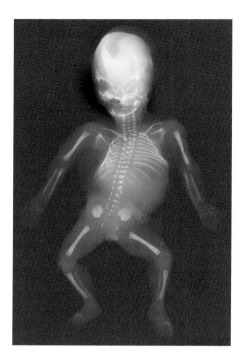

Fig. 2.31. *18th gestational week.* Fusion of neural arcs in the upper half of the thoracic spine in partial monosomy 13 q-. Microcephaly, defective ossification C1–C5. Oligodactyly; aplasia of thumb. Proximal fusion of metacarpals 4 and 5

Fig. 2.32. *18th gestational week.* Multiple vertebral segmentation defects with hemivertebrae and butterfly vertebrae in Goldenhar syndrome. Mandibular hemihypoplasia (absence of the right corpus mandibulae)

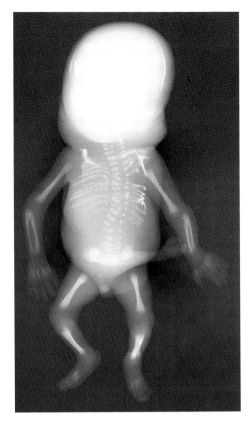

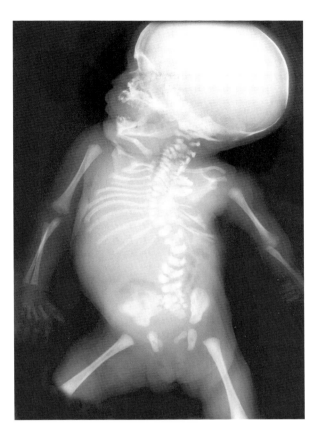

Fig. 2.33. *17th gestational week.* Multiple vertebral segmentation defects in the dorsal and upper lumbar spine in spondylothoracic dysostosis. Fusion of ribs (10 ribs on the right, 12 on the left). Short thorax. Nuchal lymphedema

Fig. 2.34. *30th gestational week.* Multiple segmentation defects of the vertebrae in MURCS association. Asymmetric vertebral aplasia/hypoplasia, left-sided rib fusions, resulting in an S-shaped scoliosis. Aplasia of the radius and right thumb

Diagnosis	Accessory radiological findings in the fetus
Acro-renal-mandibular syndrome [1] MIM 200980	Severe mandibular hypoplasia, variable and asymmetric limb reduction defects including hypoplastic or absent radius or tibia, oligodactyly, ectrodactyly, syndactyly; other defects: renal agenesis/renal dysplasia, diaphragmatic hernia
Butterfly vertebrae, isolated	Can be seen in Alagille syndrome, Aicardi syndrome
Camptomelic dysplasia [2]; see p. 114 MIM 114290	Mandibular hypoplasia; hypoplastic scapulae;, small, bell-shaped thorax; absent ribs; hypoplastic vertebrae; usually short and bowed femur and tibia; joint dislocation may include hip and radial head; absent or delayed ossification of distal femur, proximal tibia, sternum, ischium, pubis; hypoplasia of ischium and pubis; talipes equinovarus
Chromosome abnormalities [3, 4] Trisomy 13 Partial monosomy 13 q; Fig. 2.31 Trisomy 18 Triploidy	Growth retardation, hypo-ossified calvaria, hypotelorism, nuchal cystic hygroma, umbilical hernia, radial aplasia, hemivertebrae (especially fusion of the vertebral arches), coronal clefts in the lumbar spine; see Fig. 2.38

Diagnosis	Accessory radiological findings in the fetus
Diabetic embryopathy [5]; see Fig. 2.36	Hemivertebrae, absent or hypoplastic femora, hypoplastic tibia, preaxial or postaxial polydactyly, spinal dysraphism, caudal dysplasia
Dyssegmental dysplasia [6]; see p. 110 Silverman-Handmaker type [7], MIM 224410 Rolland-Desbuquois type, MIM 224400	Severe irregularity in shape and size of vertebral bodies, hypoplastic thorax with short ribs, short and wide bowed tubular long bones with wide metaphyses (dumbbell shaped), hypoplasia of basilar portions of ilia, broad and thick ischium and pubis
Fetal alcohol syndrome [8]	Intrauterine growth retardation, microcephaly vertebral segmentation defects, Klippel-Feil anomaly, reduction deformity of upper extremities, hypoplasia/aplasia of ulna, tetradactyly, clubfoot
Klippel-Feil syndrome [9]; MIM 148900	Spectrum of cervical and upper thoracic spinal fusions; hemivertebrae and occipitoatlantal fusion; Sprengel deformity; spina bifida; may be a part of Mayer-Rokitansky-Küster syndrome, MURCS association (Fig. 2.34), alcohol embryopathy, Duane anomaly-radial defects, or Goldenhar syndrome (Fig. 2.32)
Limb/pelvis hypoplasia/aplasia syndrome [10] Al-Awadi/Raas-Rothschild syndrome, MIM 276820 May be the same as Schinzel phocomelia MIM 268300	Variable and possibly asymmetric lower limb deficiency including primarily femur, tibia and fibula; absent toes; upper limb defects include absent/hypoplastic radius, ulna, carpals, metacarpals, and phalanges; radio-humeral synostosis; hypoplastic pelvis including irregular pubis, ischium; hip dislocation; thoracic involvement including wide or fused ribs, pectus carinatum
Jarcho-Levin syndrome [11]; MIM 277300 Fig. 2.33 Spondylocostal dysostosis; spondylothoracic dysostosis	Severe vertebral defects including block vertebrae; butterfly vertebrae; hemivertebrae; ribs that: have sagittal clefts with malsegmentation including fusion, are bifid, are absent or hypoplastic, appear "fan-like" or "crab-like"; spinal dysraphism; neural tube defects; congenital heart defects; and other visceral anomalies frequently reported
Lethal multiple pterygium syndrome [12] MIM 253290 X-linked lethal multiple pterygium syndrome [13] MIM 312150	Fusion of cervical vertebrae, hypoplastic scapulae, wide ribs, contractures of large joints with pterygia formation, radio-ulnar synostosis, camptodactyly of fingers, talipes equinovarus; other features: cystic hygroma and hydrops fetalis, diaphragmatic hernia
MURCS association [14]; MIM 601076 Fig. 2.34	Acronym of associated malformations: *M*ullerian duct aplasia/hypoplasia, *r*enal aplasia/ectopia, *c*ervical *s*omite (spinal) dysplasia, and upper limb defects
*O*mphalocele-*e*xstrophy of the bladder-*i*mperforate anus-*s*pinal defect (OEIS) complex [15] MIM 258040	Hemivertebrae, absent sacrum, widely spaced pubic bones, spinal dysraphism, talipes equinovarus
Spinal dysraphism	Vertebral segmentation defects (such defects also part of Arnold-Chiari II malformation, hydrocephalus)

Diagnosis	Accessory radiological findings in the fetus
Urorectal septum malformation sequence [16]	Vertebral fusion, hemivertebrae, extra or missing ribs, absent or hypoplastic sacrum, hypoplastic radius, absent or hypoplastic thumb; other defects: megacystis ("prune belly"), anal atresia, esophageal atresia, tracheoesophageal fistula, cardiac defect, renal agenesis or dysplasia, absent or ambiguous external genitalia
VATER Association [17] MIM 192350 VACTERL Association	Vertebral fusion, hemivertebrae, missing or extra ribs, rib fusion, absent or hypoplastic radius, absent or hypoplastic thumb, triphalangeal thumb, preaxial polydactyly, other limb deficiencies less commonly; other defects: anal atresia, esophageal atresia, tracheoesophageal fistula, cardiac defect, renal agenesis or dysplasia
VATER Association with hydrocephalus [18] MIM 276950, 314390	Macrocephaly secondary to hydrocephalus, hydranencephaly, vertebral fusion, hemivertebrae, missing or extra ribs, rib fusion, absent or hypoplastic radius, absent or hypoplastic thumb, triphalangeal thumb, pre-axial polydactyly, other limb deficiencies less commonly; other defects: anal atresia, esophageal atresia, tracheoesophageal fistula, cardiac defect, renal agenesis or dysplasia

References

1. Halal F, Desgranges M-F, Leduc B et al (1980) Acro-renal–mandibular syndrome. Am J Med Genet 5:277–284
2. Houston CS, Opitz JM, Spranger JW et al (1983) The campomelic syndrome: review, report of 17 cases, and follow-up on the currently 17-year-old boy first reported by Maroteaux et al in 1971. Am J Med Genet 15:3–28
3. James AE Jr, Merz T, Janower ML et al (1971) Radiological features of the most common autosomal disorders: trisomy 21–22 (mongolism or Down's syndrome), trisomy 18, trisomy 13–15, and the cri du chat syndrome. Clin Radiol 22:417–433
4. Kjaer I, Keeling JW, Hansen BF (1996) Pattern of malformations in the axial skeleton in human trisomy 18 fetuses. Am J Med Genet 65:332–336
5. Passarge E, Lenz W (1966) Syndrome of caudal regression in infants of diabetic mothers: observations of further cases. Pediatrics 37:672–675
6. Aleck KA, Grix A, Clericuzio C et al (1987) Dyssegmental dysplasias: clinical, radiographic, and morphologic evidence of heterogeneity. Am J Med Genet 7:295–312
7. Handmaker SD, Robinson LD, Campbell JA et al (1977) Dyssegmental dwarfism: a new syndrome of lethal dwarfism. Birth Defects Orig Art Ser 13:79–90
8. Herrmann J, Pallister PD, Opitz JM (1980) Tetraectrodactyly, and other skeletal manifestations in the fetal alcohol syndrome. Eur J Pediatr 133:221–226
9. Clarke RA, Catalan G, Diwan AD, Kearsley JH (1998) Heterogeneity in Klippel-Feil syndrome: a new classification. Pediatr Radiol 28:967–974
10. Raas-Rothschild A, Goodman RM, Meyer S et al (1988) Pathological features and prenatal diagnosis in the newly-recognized limb/pelvis-hypoplasia/aplasia syndrome. J Med Genet 25:687–697
11. Jarcho S, Levin PM (1938) Hereditary malformation of the vertebral bodies. Bull Johns Hopkins Hosp 62:216
12. Hall JG (1984) Editorial comment: the lethal multiple pterygia syndromes. Am J Med Genet 17:803–807
13. Tolmie JL, Patrick A, Yates JRW (1987) A lethal multiple pterygium syndrome with apparent X-linked recessive inheritance. Am J Med Genet 27:913–919
14. Greene RA, Bloch MJ, Shuff DS, Iozzo RV (1986) MURCS association with additional congenital anomalies. Hum Pathol 17:88–91
15. Carey JC, Greenbaum, B, Hall BD (1978) The OEIS Complex (omphalocele, exstrophy, imperforate anus, spinal defects). Birth Defects Orig Art Ser 14:253–263
16. Wheeler PG, Weaver DD, Obeime MO et al (1997) Urorectal septum malformation sequence: report of thirteen additional cases and review of the literature. Am J Med Genet 73:456–462
17. Quan L, Smith DW (1972) The VATER association: vertebral defects, anal atresia, tracheoesophageal fistula with esophageal atresia, radial dysplasia. Birth Defects Orig Art Ser 8:75–78
18. Iafolla AK, McConkie-Rosell A, Chen YT (1991) VATER and hydrocephalus: distinct syndrome? Am J Med Genet 38:46–51

Pelvic-Sacral Abnormalities

Sacral Agenesis/Hypogenesis/Caudal Dysplasia; Pubic Bone Dysgenesisa

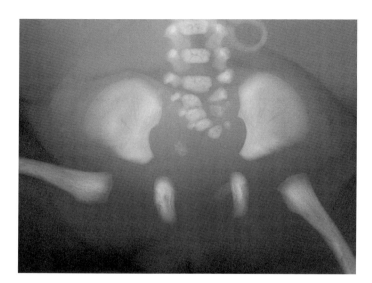

Fig. 2.35. *34th gestational week.* Semilunar dysostosis of the sacrum (scimitar shape) due to an anterior meningocele. (Currarino triad)

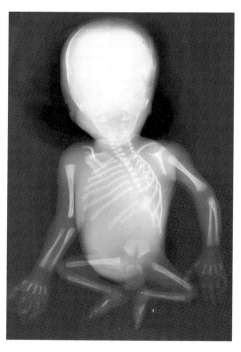

Fig. 2.36. *22nd gestational week.* Aplasia of the lower spine in Diabetic embryopathy. Posterior, fork-like fusion of the 8th and 9th ribs, partial fusion of iliac bones, narrow pelvis. Slender tibia and fibula due to hypokinesia. Stippled ossification of calcaneus

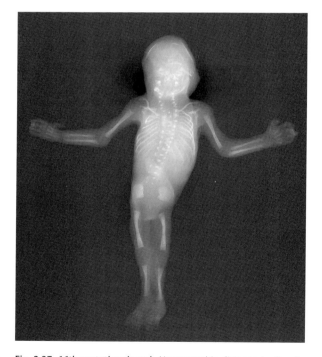

Fig. 2.37. *16th gestational week.* Narrow pubic distance in dipodic sirenomelia. Multiple vertebral segmentation defects and fusion of neural arches. Desmal fusion of lower legs. Mirroring of shanks and feet (tibia and hallux on the outside). Sacrum not ossified, narrow ossa ischii

Diagnosis	Accessory radiological findings in the fetus
Achondrogenesis, type II; see p. 106 Hypochondrogenesis MIM 200600 Lethal type II collagenopathies [1] MIM 200610	Absent or severely delayed ossification of vertebral bodies, short and horizontally oriented ribs, absent or delayed ossification of pubic and ischial bones, small iliac bones with concave borders, small scapulae, very short long bones with cupped metaphyses, fetal hydrops
Boomerang dysplasia[a] [2]; see p. 148 MIM 112310	Similar to atelosteogenesis I, but more severe; hypo-ossification of calvarium; relative macrocephaly; micrognathia; absent or severely retarded ossification of vertebral bodies; long clavicles with normal ossification; narrow interpedicular distance of the thoracic spine with widening in the lumbar spine; very short and deformed long tubular bones (the femur may be fan- or boomerang-shaped); absent pubic ossification centers; hydrops fetalis
Camptomelic dysplasia[a] [3]; see p. 114 MIM 211970	Mandibular hypoplasia; hypoplastic scapulae; small bell-shaped thorax; absent ribs; hypoplastic vertebrae; usually short and bowed femur and tibia; joint dislocation may include hip and radial head; absent or delayed ossification of distal femur, proximal tibia, sternum, ischium, pubis; hypoplasia of ischium and pubis; talipes equinovarus
Cleidocranial dysostosis [4] MIM 119600	Partially absent clavicles, delayed ossification of the pubic bones, cleft mandible, cleft palate
Currarino triad [5, 6]; MIM 176450 Fig. 2.35	Sickle-shaped sacrum, presacral mass, anterior meningocele
Diabetic embryopathy [7]; Fig. 2.36	Hemivertebrae, absent or hypoplastic femora, hypoplastic tibiae, preaxial or postaxial polydactyly, spinal dysraphism, rib fusion in the midline
Axial mesodermal dysplasia spectrum [8]	Caudal dysplasia, hemivertebrae, scoliosis, absent or bifid ribs, lower limb contractures, talipes equinovarus, hemifacial microsomia
Isolated defect [9]	Variable lumbar vertebral agenesis; fused iliac wings; lower limb contractures with pterygia; hypoplasia of femur, tibia, fibula; talipes equinovarus
Limb-body wall complex [10]; MIM 217100 see Fig. 2.15	Defect of lower abdominal wall, bladder exstrophy, pubic diastasis, segmental defects of lower extremities, spinal segmentation defects
Limb/pelvis hypoplasia/aplasia syndrome [11] Schinzel phocomelia syndrome MIM 268300 May be the same as Al-Awadi/Raas-Rothschild syndrome MIM 276820	Parieto-occipital skull defect, femoral hypoplasia, absent ulnae and fibulae, radial agenesis, oligodactyly, preaxial polydactyly, diaphragmatic hernia
Omphalocele-Exstrophy of the bladder-Imperforate anus-Spinal defect (OEIS) complex[a] [12] MIM 258040	Hemivertebrae, widely spaced pubic bones, spinal dysraphism, talipes equinovarus

Diagnosis	Accessory radiological findings in the fetus
Opsismodysplasia[a] [13] MIM 258480	Delayed skeletal maturation, shortening of hand bones, rhizomelic shortening of limbs, severe platyspondyly, absent ossification of vertebrae, narrow thorax, delayed ossification of ischiopubic bones
Pubic distance, extended[a] see Fig. 2.15	Hint of an underlying epispadia, bladder exstrophy, ventral wall defect; syndromatic or non-syndromatic
Pubic distance, narrow[a] see Fig. 2.13	Hint of an underlying urethral aplasia/atresia, prune belly syndrome; syndromatic or non-syndromatic
Schinzel-Giedion syndrome[a] [14] MIM 269150	Sclerosis of the base of the skull and midface, gap in the occipital bone, broad ribs, mesomelia of upper limbs with bowing of its long bones
Sirenomelia [15]; Fig. 2.37 MIM 182940	Hemivertebrae, fusion of vertebrae, bifid or fused ribs, spinal dysraphism, single or fused lower limb with single or fused femora and tibiae, variable foot abnormalities depending on degree of fusion, sometimes both tibiae and fibulae rotated by 180 degrees, hypoplastic/absent radius
Spondyloepiphyseal dysplasia congenita[a] [1, 16]; see p. 108 MIM 183900 Spondylometepiphyseal dysplasia (Strudwick)[a] [17, 18] MIM 271668	Short trunk, short limbs; similar radiologic signs of both diseases during fetal period; growth retardation, ovoid vertebrae; no ossification of pubic rami
Urorectal septum malformation sequence[a] [19]	Hemivertebrae, hypoplasia of femur and/or tibia, talipes equinovarus, polydactyly, radial agenesis, megacystis ("prune belly")
VATER Associationa [20] MIM 192350 VACTERL Association; see Figs. 2.9, 2.13	Vertebral fusion, hemivertebrae, missing or extra ribs, rib fusion, absent or hypoplastic radius, absent or hypoplastic thumb, triphalangeal thumb, preaxial polydactyly, other limb deficiencies less common; other defects include anal atresia, esophageal atresia, tracheoesophageal fistula, cardiac defect, renal agenesis or dysplasia

[a] Syndromes with pubic bone dysgenesis.

References

1. Spranger J, Winterpacht A, Zabel B (1994) The type II collagenopathies: a spectrum of chondrodysplasias. Eur J Pediatr 153 : 56–65
2. Winship I, Cremin B, Beighton P (1990) Boomerang dysplasia. Am J Med Genet 36 : 440–443
3. Houston CS, Opitz JM, Spranger JW et al (1983) The campomelic syndrome: review, report of 17 cases, and follow-up on the currently 17-year-old boy first reported by Maroteaux et al in 1971. Am J Med Genet 15 : 3–28
4. Cooper Sc, Flaitz CM, Johnston DA, Lee B Hecht JT (2001) A natural history of cleidocranial dysplasia. Am J Med Genet 104 : 1–6
5. Currarino G, Coln D, Votteler T (1981) Triad of anorectal, sacral, and presacral anomalies. Am J Roentgenol 137 : 395–398
6. Ross AJ, Ruiz-Perez V, Wang Y et al (1998) A homeobox gene, HLXB9, is the major locus for dominantly inherited sacral agenesis. Nature Genet 20 : 358–361
7. Passarge E, Lenz W (1966) Syndrome of caudal regression in infants of diabetic mothers: observations of further cases. Pediatrics 37 : 672–675
8. Russell LJ, Weaver DD, Bull MJ (1981) The axial mesodermal dysplasia spectrum. Pediatrics 67 : 176–182
9. Renshaw TS (1978) Sacral agenesis: a classification and review of twenty-three cases. J Bone Joint Surg Am 60 : 373–383
10. Higginbottom MC, Jones KL, Hall BD (1979) The amniotic band disruption complex: timing of amniotic rupture and variable spectra of consequent defects. J Pediatr 95 : 544–549
11. Chitayat D, Stalker HJ, Vekemans M et al (1993) Phocomelia, oligodactyly, and acrania: the Schinzel-phocomelia syndrome. Am J Med Genet 45 : 297–299
12. Carey JC, Greenbaum B, Hall BD (1978) The OEIS Complex (omphalocele, exstrophy, imperforate anus, spinal defects). Birth Defects Orig Art Ser 14 : 253–263

13. Maroteaux P, Stanescu V, Stanescu R et al (1984) Opsismodyspla-sia: a new type of chondrodysplasia with predominant involve-ment of the bones of the hand and the vertebrae. Am J Med Genet 19:171–182

14. Labrune P, Lyonnet S, Zupan V et al (1994) Three new cases of the Schinzel-Giedion syndrome and review of the literature. Am J Med Genet 50:90–93

15. Duhamel B (1961) From the mermaid to anal imperforation: the syndrome of caudal regression. Arch Dis Child 36:152–155

16. Shebib SM, Chudley AE, Reed MH (1991) Spondylometepiphyseal dysplasia congenita, Strudwick type. Pediatr Radiol 21:298–300

17. Spranger JW, Langer LO Jr (1970) Spondyloepiphyseal dysplasia congenita. Radiology 94:313–322

18. Spranger JW, Maroteaux P (1983) Genetic heterogeneity of spon-dyloepiphyseal dysplasia congenita? Am J Med Genet 14:601–602

19. Wheeler PG, Weaver DD, Obeime MO et al (1997) Urorectal sep-tum malformation sequence: report of thirteen additional cases and review of the literature. Am J Med Genet 73:456–462

20. Quan L, Smith DW (1972) The VATER association: vertebral defects, anal atresia, tracheoesophageal fistula with esophageal atresia, radial dysplasia. Birth Defects Orig Art Ser 8:75–78

Coronal Clefts of Vertebral Bodies

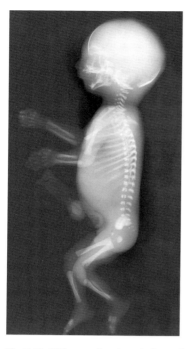

Fig. 2.38. *18th gestational week.* Coronal clefts of the thoracic and lumbar vertebral bodies in Trisomy 21. Otherwise normal skeleton

Diagnosis	Accessory radiological findings in the fetus
See Atelosteogenesis I [1–3] and related osteochondrodysplasias; see p. 148 MIM 108720, 108721, 112310	Hypoplastic vertebral bodies, especially of cervical and thoracic spine; hypoplastic and tapered (distal) humerus and femur; bowed radius, ulna, tibia; absent or hypoplastic fibula; absent or hypo-ossified metacarpals and phalanges
Chondrodysplasia punctata, rhizomelic type [4, 5]; see p. 142 MIM 215100	Punctate calcifications primarily around the ends of long bones, hypoplasia of humerus and femur, wide or splayed metaphyses, platyspondyly
Chondrodysplasia punctata, tibia-metacarpal type [6]; MIM 118651	Stippling of sacrum and carpals; dislocation of hip, knee, elbow; short femur, tibia, metacarpals, phalanges; asymmetry
Chromosome abnormalities Trisomy 13 [7] Trisomy 18 [8] Trisomy 21 [9]; Fig. 2.38 Triploidy [10]	Besides the other signs (such as growth retardation, hypo-ossified calvaria, hypotelorism, nuchal cystic hygroma, umbilical hernia, radius aplasia), hemivertebrae (especially fusion of the vertebral arches), coronal clefts in the lumbar spine
Desbuquois syndrome [11, 12]; see p. 146 MIM 251540	Mild platyspondyly, hypoplasia of the ilia (base), short femoral neck and greater trochanter ("monkey wrench" appearance), mild shortening of long bones with flared metaphyses, multiple large and small joint dislocations, advanced carpal and tarsal ossification, accessory ossification centers of metacarpals and metatarsals (digits I and II)

Diagnosis	Accessory radiological findings in the fetus
Fibrochondrogenesis [13, 14]; see p. 101 MIM 228520	Micrognathia; absent or hypo-ossification of vertebral bodies, especially posteriorly; platyspondyly; short ribs with splayed ends; short, broad ilia with basilar spurs, short long tubular bones with metaphyseal flaring ("dumbbell-shaped")
Lethal Kniest-like dysplasia [15], MIM 245190 Kniest dysplasia [16], MIM156550; see p. 108	Relative macrocephaly, micrognathia, platyspondyly, broad ilia with hypoplasia of the base, short tubular bones with wide metaphyses, short femoral neck, hydrops fetalis
Short rib-polydactyly syndrome, type I (Saldino-Noonan) [17]; see p. 133 MIM 263530	Relative macrocephaly, very short horizontal ribs, hypoplasia of scapula, small ilia, very short femur and humerus with pointed ends, absent or hypo-ossification of other long tubular and short tubular bones, postaxial polydactyly, hydrops fetalis

References

1. Sillence DO, Worthington SD, Dixon J, Osborn R, Kozlowski K (1997) Atelosteogenesis syndromes: a review with comments on their pathogenesis. Pediatr Radiol 27 : 388–396
2. Hunter AGW, Carpenter BF (1991) Atelosteogenesis I and boomerang dysplasia: a question of nosology. Clin Genet 39 : 471–480
3. Winship I, Cremin B, Beighton P (1990) Boomerang dysplasia. Am J Med Genet 36 : 440–443
4. Gilbert EF, Iopitz JM, Spranger JW et al (1976) Chondrodysplasia punctata, rhizomelic form: pathological and radiologic studies in three infants. Eur J Pediatr 123 : 89–109
5. Poulos A, Sheffield L, Sharp P et al (1988) Rhizomelic chondrodysplasia punctata: clinical, pathologic and biochemical findings in two patients. J Pediatr 113 : 685–690
6. Rittler M, Menger H, Spranger J (1990) Chondrodysplasia punctata, tibia-metacarpal (MT) type. Am J Med Genet 37 : 200–208
7. Kjær I, Keeling JW, Hansen BF (1997) Pattern of malformations in the axial skeleton in human trisomy 13 fetuses. Am J Med Genet 70 : 421–426
8. Kjær I, Keeling JW, Hansen BF (1996) Pattern of malformations in the axial skeleton in human trisomy 18 fetuses. Am J Med Genet 65 : 332–336
9. Keeling JW, Hansen BF, Kjær I (1997) Pattern of malformations in the axial skeleton in human trisomy 21 fetuses. Am J Med Genet 68 : 466–471
10. Kjær I, Keeling JW, Smith NM, Hansen BF (1997) Pattern of malformations in the axial skeleton in human triploid fetuses. Am J Med Genet 72 : 216–221
11. Desbuquois G, Grenier B, Michel J et al (1966) Nanisme chondrodystrophique avec ossification anarchique et polymalformations chez deux soeurs. Arch Fr Pediatr 23 : 573–587
12. Shohat M, Lachman R, Gruber HE et al (1994) Desbuquois syndrome: clinical, radiographic, and morphologic characterization. Am J Med Genet 52 : 9–18
13. Whitley CB, Langer LO Jr, Ophoven J et al (1984) Fibrochondrogenesis: lethal, autosomal recessive chondrodysplasia with distinctive cartilage histopathology. Am J Med Genet 19 : 265–275
14. Al-Gazali LI, Bakalinova D, Bakir M et al (1997) Fibrochondrogenesis: clinical and radiological features. Clin Dysmorphol 6 : 157–163
15. Sconyers SM, Rimoin DL, Lachman RS et al (1983) A distinct chondrodysplasia resembling 15 Kniest dysplasia: clinical, roentgenographic, histologic, and ultrasound findings. J Pediatr 103 : 898–904
16. Freisinger P, Bonaventure J, Stoess H et al (1996) Type II collagenopathies: are there additional family members? Am J Med Genet 63 : 137–143
17. Saldino RM, Noonan CD (1972) Severe thoracic dystrophy with striking micromelia, abnormal osseous development, including the spine, and multiple visceral anomalies. Am J Roentgenol 114 : 257–263

Ectopia Cordis

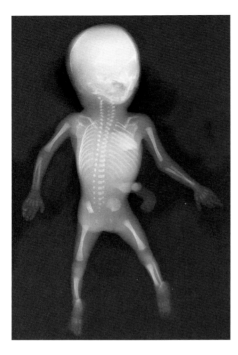

Fig. 2.39. *18th gestational week.* Body wall defect: ectopic heart in pentalogy of Cantrell. The shadow of the ectopic heart projects onto the upper part of the left hemithorax. Slender abdomen. Otherwise normal

Diagnosis	Accessory radiological findings in the fetus
Amniotic band disruption sequence [1, 2]; ADAM complex (*A*mniotic *D*eformity, *A*dhesions, *M*utilations) Limb-body wall complex MIM 217100	Usually asymmetric transverse terminal limb reductions/amputations and variable terminal syndactyly/pseudosyndactyly; may also include oligodactyly, hypoplasia of long bones, craniofacial and ventral wall disruption.
Pentalogy of Cantrell [3] Thoracoabdominal syndrome; MIM 313850 Fig. 2.39	Sternal defects including agenesis, clefting or bifid sternum, absence of lower third of sternum; other defects include supraumbilical midline defect (omphalocele), central diaphragmatic hernia, pericardial defect, congenital heart defect
Sternal malformation-vascular dysplasia association [4] Sternal clefts-telangiectasia/hemangiomas Hemangiomas – midline abdominal raphe [5] MIM 140850	Absent or bifid sternum, pectus excavatum, absent or hypoplastic clavicles; micrognathia, cleft mandible; other features include midline hemangiomas of face and/or chest, midline supraumbilical raphe

References

1. Beiber FR, Mostoufi-Zadeh M, Birnholz JC (1984) Amniotic band sequence associated with ectopia cordis in one twin. J Pediatr 105:817–819

2. Kaplan LC, Matsuoka R, Gilbert EF et al (1985) Ectopia cordis and cleft sternum: evidence for mechanical teratogenesis following rupture of the chorion or yolk sac. Am J Med Genet 21:187–199

3. Cantrell JR, Haller JA, Ravitsch MA (1958) A syndrome of congenital defects involving the abdominal wall, sternum, diaphragm, pericardium and heart. Surg Gynecol Obstet 107:602–614

4. Hersh JH, Waterfill D, Rutledge J et al (1985) Sternal malformation/vascular dysplasia association. Am J Med Genet 21:177–186

5. Geller JD, Topper SF, Hashimoto K (1991) Diffuse neonatal hemangiomatosis: a new constellation of findings. J Am Acad Dermatol 24:816–818

Ventral Wall Defects/Omphalocele/Gastroschisis

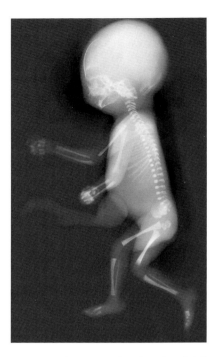

Fig. 2.40. *24th gestational week.* Body wall defect: omphalocele in trisomy 18. Deficient ossification of calvaria. The 2nd digit of the right hand overlaps the 3rd

Diagnosis	Accessory radiological findings in the fetus
Amniotic band disruption sequence ADM complex (*Amniotic Deformity, Adhesions, Mutilations*) Limb-body wall complex [1]; MIM 217100 see Fig. 2.15	Usually asymmetric transverse terminal limb reductions/amputations and variable terminal syndactyly/pseudosyndactyly; may also include oligodactyly, hypoplasia of long bones, craniofacial and ventral wall disruption
Boomerang dysplasia [2, 3]; see p. 148 MIM 112310	Similar to atelosteogenesis I, but more severe; hypoossification of calvarium; relative macrocephaly; micrognathia; absent or severely retarded ossification of vertebral bodies; long clavicles with normal ossification; narrow interpedicular distance of the thoracic spine with widening in the lumbar spine; very short and deformed long tubular bones (the femur may be fan- or boomerang-shaped); hydrops fetalis
Chromosome abnormality, trisomy 13 [4]	Microcephaly, hypotelorism, small orbits, hypo-ossification of calvarium, spinal dysraphism, hemivertebrae, absent/supernumerary/fused ribs, hypoplasia of pelvis, oligodactyly, polydactyly, syndactyly, camptodactyly, vertical talus; other defects: heart abnormalities, omphalocele, holoprosencephaly, neural tube defect, cystic hygroma, hydrops fetalis

Diagnosis	Accessory radiological findings in the fetus
Chromosome abnormality, trisomy 18 [4, 5]; Fig. 2.40	Microcephaly, hypo-ossification of calvarium, hypoplasia of maxilla and/or mandible, microretrognathia, absent or thin ribs, short sternum, spinal dysraphism, hypoplasia of pelvis, hypoplasia of first metacarpal, flexion deformities and overlapping fingers, vertical talus, short first toe, hammertoes; other defects: intrauterine growth retardation, heart abnormalities, omphalocele, neural tube defect
Elejalde syndrome [6] MIM 200995	Craniosynostosis, hypertelorism, shortening of all long bones, postaxial polydactyly; other features include generalized overgrowth, cystic hygroma, hydrops fetalis.
Melnick-Needles osteodysplasty [7, 8] MIM 309350 Oto-palato-digital syndrome, type II [9, 10]; see p. 124 MIM 304120	Hypo-ossification of calvarium, sclerosis of skull base, large anterior fontanelle, micrognathia, thin/wavy/beaded ribs with irregular cortex, hypoplastic scapula, flared ilia with hypoplastic base, kyphosis, scoliosis, lordosis, S-shaped bowing of long bones, metaphyseal flaring, coxa valga, genus valga, short distal phalanges, absent or hypoplastic metacarpals and metatarsals, absent or hypoplastic thumb and/or hallux; other defects: urinary obstruction, multiple joint dislocations
Omphalocele-exstrophy of the cloaca-imperforate anus-spinal defect (OEIS complex) [11] MIM 258040	Absent or hypoplastic sacrum, hemivertebrae, scoliosis, spinal dysraphism, pubic diastasis, talipes equinovarus
Pseudotrisomy 13 syndrome [12, 13] MIM 264480	Microcephaly, micrognathia, hemivertebrae, absent or hypoplastic radius or ulna, postaxial polydactyly, preaxial polydactyly, absent or hypoplastic tibia, broad hallux, talipes equinovarus
Short rib-polydactyly, Beemer-Langer type [14]; see p. 134 MIM 269860	Short horizontal ribs, short tubular bones, tibia short but longer than fibula, bowed radius and ulna, preaxial or postaxial polydactyly, hypoplastic ilia; other defects: CNS abnormalities, cleft lip, heart, kidneys, hydrops fetalis
Thoracoabdominal syndrome Pentalogy of Cantrell [15, 16] MIM 313850	Short, cleft or bifid sternum, central/anterior diaphragmatic hernia; other defects include ectopia cordis, congenital heart defect

References

1. Jones KL, Smith DW, Hall BW et al (1974) A pattern of craniofacial and limb defects secondary to aberrant tissue bands. J Pediatr 84:90–95
2. Hunter AGW, Carpenter BF (1991) Atelosteogenesis I and boomerang dysplasia: a question of nosology. Clin Genet 39:471–480
3. Winship I, Cremin B, Beighton P (1990) Boomerang dysplasia. Am J Med Genet 36:440–443
4. James AE Jr, Merz T, Janower ML et al (1971) Radiological features of the most common autosomal disorders: trisomy 21–22 (mongolism or Down's syndrome), trisomy 18, trisomy 13–15, and the cri du chat syndrome. Clin Radiol 22:417–433

5. Franceschini P, Fabris C, Ponzone A et al (1974) Skeletal alterations in Edwards' disease (trisomy 18 syndrome). Ann Radiol (Paris) 17:361–367
6. Elejalde BR, Giraldo C, Jimenez R et al (1977) Acrocephalopolydactylous dysplasia. Birth Defects Orig Art Ser 13:53–67
7. Donnenfeld AE, Conrad KA, Roberts NS et al (1987) Melnick-Needles syndromes in males: a lethal multiple congenital anomalies syndrome. Am J Med Genet 27:159–173
8. Von Oeyen P, Holmes LB, Trelstad RL et al (1982) Omphalocele and multiple severe congenital anomalies associated with osteodysplasty (Melnick-Needles syndrome). Am J Med Genet 13:453–463

9. Young K, Barth CK, Moore C et al (1993) Otopalatodigital syndrome type II associated with omphalocele: report of three cases. Am J Med Genet 45:481–487

10. Verloes A, Lesenfants S, Barr M et al (2000) Fronto-otopalatodigital osteodysplasia: clinical evidence for a single entity encompassing Melnick-Needles syndrome, otopalatodigital syndromes types 1 and 2, and frontometaphyseal dysplasia. Am J Med Genet 90:407–422

11. Carey JC, Greenbaum B, Hall BD (1978) The OEIS complex (omphalocele, exstrophy, imperforate anus, spinal defects). Birth Defects Orig Art Ser 14:253–263

12. Cohen MM Jr, Gorlin RJ (1991) Pseudo-trisomy 13 syndrome. Am J Med Genet 39:332–335

13. Boles RG, Teebi AS, Neilson KA et al (1992) Pseudo-trisomy 13 syndrome with upper limb shortness and radial hypoplasia. Am J Med Genet 44:638–640

14. Beemer FA, Langer LO Jr, Klep-de Pater JM et al (1983) A new short rib syndrome: report of two cases. Am J Med Genet 14:115–123

15. Cantrell JR, Haller JA, Ravitsch MA (1958) A syndrome of congenital defects involving the abdominal wall, sternum, diaphragm, pericardium and heart. Surg Gynecol Obstet 107:602–614

16. Carmi R, Barbash A, Mares AJ (1990) Thoracoabdominal syndrome (TAS): a new X-linked dominant disorder. Am J Med Genet 36:109–114

3 The Osteochondrodysplasias

Introduction

The presence of widespread, often symmetric, skeletal abnormalities raises the possibility of a generalized skeletal dysplasia. Osteochondrodysplasias are structural or formative defects that continue to evolve after blastogenesis, i.e., approximately the 8th gestational week. At this time, the patterning of individual bones as organs, i.e., of the single constituents of the axial skeleton and limbs, is complete. Many genes involved in the early patterning and development of the skeleton are no longer expressed. On the other hand, defects of growth, maturation, and homeostasis may continue to manifest until adulthood and thereafter, producing abnormalities recognizable by the histologic study of chondroosseous tissue.

In this book only osteochondrodysplasias manifesting during fetal life are depicted. Many of them are lethal. Their recognition in utero and differentiation from early-manifesting nonlethal osteochondrodysplasias by sonography is difficult and has been the subject of many studies (Avni et al. 1996; Doray et al. 2000; Rouse et al. 1990; Spirt et al. 1990; Tretter et al. 1998). Postnatally, anterio-posterior and lateral radiographs of the entire fetus and of selected sites, notably the hands, often allow for a specific diagnosis with only a limited number of differential diagnoses. In that respect the conditions presented here differ from those in Chap. 2 of the book which occur less specifically in a great number of diseases.

More fetal osteochondrodysplasias exist than are illustrated in this book. Some of them may be variant expressions of known dysplasias. Other represent bona fide entities waiting for future delineation (e.g., Akaba et al. 1996; Al Gazali et al. 1996; Brodie et al. 1999; Goldblatt 1998; Kerner et al. 1998; Khosravi et al. 1998; Kozlowski et al. 1995; Morton et al. 1998; Müller et al. 1992; Nishimura et al. 1998; Pinto et al. 1993; Saito et al. 1989; Saint-Martin et al. 1979; Seller et al. 1996).

References

Akaba K, Nishiumura G, Hashimoto M, Wakabayashi T, Kanasugi H, Hayasaka K (1996) New form of platyspondylic lethal chondrodysplasia. Am J Med Genet 66 : 464–467

Al Gazali LI, Devadas K, Hall CM (1996) A new lethal neonatal short limb dwarfism. Clin Dysmorphol 5 : 159–164

Avni EF, Rypens E, Zappa M, Donner C, Vanregemorter N, Cohen E (1996) Antenatal diagnosis of short-limb dwarfism: sonographic approach. Pediatr Radiol 26 : 171–178

Brodie SG, Lachman RS, McGovern MM, Mekikian PB, Wilcox WR (1999) Lethal osteosclerotic skeletal dysplasia with intracellular inclusion bodies. Am J Med Genet 83 : 372–377

Cobben JM, Cornel MC, Dijkstra I, ten Kate LP (1990) Prevalence of lethal osteochondrodysplasias. Am J Med Genet 36 : 377–378

Connor JM, Connor RAC, Sweet EM, Gibson AAM, Patrick WJA, McNay MB, Redford DHA (1986) Lethal neonatal chondrodysplasias in the West of Scotland 1970–1983. Am J Med Genet 22 : 243–253

Doray B, Favre R, Viville B, Langer B, Dreyfus M, Stoll C (2000) Prenatal sonographic diagnosis of skeletal dysplasias. A report of 47 cases. Ann Génét 43 : 163–169

Goldblatt JK, Knowles S (1989) A unique lethal spondylocostal metaphyseal dysplasia: a case report. Clin Dysmorphol 7 : 115–118

Kerner B, Rimoin DL, Lachman RS (1998) Mesomelic shortening of the upper extremities with spur formation and cutaneous dimpling. Pediatr Radiol 28 : 794–797

Khosravi M, Weaver DD, Bull M, Lachman R, Rimoin DL (1998) Lethal syndrome of skeletal dysplasia and progressive central nervous system degeneration. Am J Med Genet 77 : 63–71

Kozlowski K, John E, Masel J, Muralinath S, Vijayalakshmi G (1995) Case report: neonatal platyspondylic dwarfism – a new form. Brit J Radiol 68 : 1254–1256

Morton JEV, Kilby MD, Rushton I (1998) A new lethal autosomal recessive skeletal dysplasia with associated dysmorphic features. Clin Dysmorphol 7 : 109–114

Müller D, Kozlowski K, Sillence D (1992) Lethal micromelic facial bones sclerosis dysplasia. Br J Radiol 65 : 1137–1139

Nishimura G, Nakayama M, Fuke Y, Suchara N (1998) A lethal osteochondrodysplasia with mesomelic brachymelia, round pelvis, and congenital hepatic fibrosis: two siblings born to consanguineous parents. Pediatr Radiol 28 : 43–47

Pinto A, Hwang WS, McLeod R, Moscowitz W, Lachman RS, Rimoin DL (1993) A new variant of lethal neonatal short-limbed platyspondylic dwarfism. Arch Pathol Lab Med 117 : 322–325

Rasmussen SA, Bieber FR, Benacerraf BR, Lachman RS, Rimoin DL, Holmes LB (1996) Epidemiology of osteochondrodysplasias: changing trends due to advances in prenatal diagnosis. Am J Med Genet 61 : 49–58

Rouse GA, Filly RA, Toomey F, Grube GL (1990) Short-limb skeletal dysplasias: evaluation of the fetal spine with sonography and radiography. Radiology 174 : 177–180

Saito N, Kuba A, Tsuruta (1989) Lethal form of fibuloulnar a/hypoplasia with renal abnormalities. Am J Med Genet 32 : 452–456

Saint-Martin J, Péborde J Dupont H, Béguère A, Labs A (1979) Malformations osseuses complexes d'évolution létale. Arch Fanc Pédiat 36 : 188–193

Seller MJ, Berry AC, Maxwell D, McLennan A, Hall CM (1996) A new lethal chondrodysplasia with platyspondyly, long bone angulation and mixed bone density. Clin Dysmorphol 5 : 213–215

Spirt BA, Oliphant M, Gottlieb RH, Gordon LP (1990) Prenatal sonographic evaluation of short-limbed dwarfism: an algorithmic approach. Radiographics 10 : 217–236

Tretter AE, Saunders RC, Meyers CMK, Dungan JS, Grumbach K, Sun CCJ, Campbell AB, Wulfsberg EA (1998) Antenatal diagnosis of lethal skeletal dysplasias. Am J Med Genet 75 : 518–522

Thanatophoric Dysplasia I   MIM 187600

Synonym: Thanatophoric Dwarfism I. Includes San Diego variant of platyspondylic chondrodysplasia.

Major Radiographic Features:
- Enlarged skull; rarely craniosynostosis with cloverleaf formation
- Narrow thorax due to short ribs
- Flattened vertebral bodies with central depression of upper and lower plates in most cases; wafer-thin vertebral bodies in San Diego variant
- Hypoplastic iliac wings with horizontal inferior margins, often medially extending radiolucent band or multiple ossification centers in inferiolateral aspects of ilia, narrow sacrosciatic notches, unossified pubic bones
- Short, broad, and bowed tubular bones with flared metaphyses
- Rounded, radiolucent appearance of proximal femoral end in most cases; squared proximal end with ragged metaphyseal margin in San Diego variant
- Very short and broad tubular bones of hands and feet

Mode of Inheritance: Autosomal dominant.

Molecular Basis: Various mutations of the *FGFR3* gene encoding the fibroblast growth factor receptor 3.

Prenatal Diagnosis: Ultrasound diagnosis in the 2nd trimester can be confirmed by mutation analysis of *FGFR3* in cultured amniotic cells or cord blood cells.

Differential Diagnosis: *Thanatophoric dysplasia II* differs by having straight tubular bones and more frequent occurrence of craniosynostosis with cloverleaf formation.

The appearance of the vertebral bodies, pelvis, and tubular bones rules out other lethal chondrodysplasias including the various types of *achondrogenesis* and *Schneckenbecken dysplasias* with which thanatophoric dysplasia has been confused. A radiologically similar disease with good prognosis is *achondroplasia*. The bone changes in that disorder are similar but milder than those in thanatophoric dysplasia.

Prognosis: Most patients are stillborn or die shortly after birth from cardiorespiratory failure. With appropriate life support a few patients are known to have survived beyond the age of 9 years, but show growth failure, severe mental and motor deficiency due to structural brain abnormalities, and prolonged dependency on ventilator assistance.

Remarks: The San Diego variant characterized by wafer-thin vertebral bodies, less severely bowed long tubular bones with ragged metaphyseal margins and absence of the gland-like radiolucency of the upper femoral end, and formerly thought to represent a distinct entity called "San Diego type of platyspondylic chondrodysplasia," has been shown to be caused be the same mutations that cause thanatophoric dysplasia I.

References

Bakter KM, Olson Ds, Harding CO, Pauli RM (1997) Long-term survival in typical thanatophoric dysplasia type 1. Am J Med Genet 70: 427–436

Brodie SG, Kitoh H, Lachman RS, Nolasco LM, Mekikian P, Wilcox WR (1999) Platyspondylic lethal skeletal dysplasia, San Diego type, is caused by FGF3 mutations. Am J Med Genet 84:476–480

Chen CP, Chern SR, Shih JC, Wang W, Yeh LF, Chang TY, Tzen CY (2001) Prenatal diagnosis and genetic analysis of type I and type II thanatophoric dysplasia. Prenat Diagn 21:89–95

Spranger JW, Brill PWE, Poznanski A (2002) Bone dysplasia, 2nd edn., Elsevier GmbH, Urban & Fischer, Munich

Wilcox WR, Tavormina PL, Krakow D, Kitoh H, Lachman RS, Wasmut JJ, Thompson LM, Rimoin DL (1998) Molecular, radiologic, and histopathologic correlations in thanatophoric dysplasia. Am J Med Genet 78:274–278

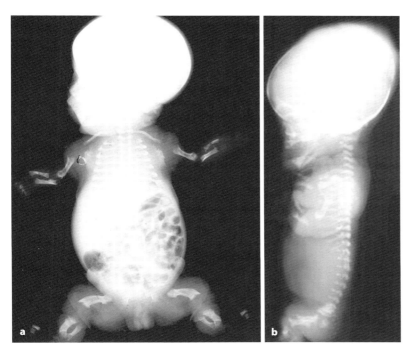

Fig. 3.1a, b. *Thanatophoric dysplasia I.* Newborn, 37 weeks' gestation. **a** Prominent features are narrow thorax, flat vertebral bodies, squared iliac wings with wide, horizontal inferior margins, short and broad tubular bones, curved femora with radiolucent upper ends. **b** The vertebral bodies are flattened, the posterior elements are well developed. (From: Spranger et al.: Bone Dysplasias, 2nd edn., 2002, with kind permission from Elsevier GmbH, Urban & Fischer, Munich)

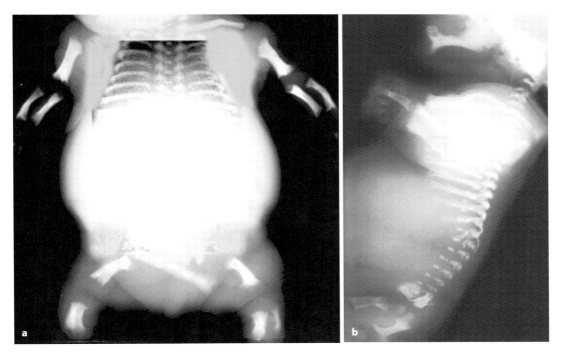

Fig. 3.2a, b. *Thanatophoric dysplasia I, San Diego variant.* Newborn, 38 weeks' gestation. **a** Compared to Fig. 1, the tubular bones are also short and broad, but the femora are only minimally bowed. **b** The vertebral bodies are wafer thin. The patient did not have a cloverleaf skull

Thanatophoric Dysplasia II   MIM 187601

Synonym: Thanatophoric dysplasia with Kleeblattschädel (cloverleaf skull).

Major Radiographic Features:
- Often craniosynostosis with cloverleaf formation
- Narrow thorax due to short ribs
- Flattened vertebral bodies with irregular upper and lower end plates
- Hypoplastic iliac wings with horizontal inferior margins, often medially extending radiolucent band or multiple ossification centers in inferiolateral aspects of ilia, narrow sacrosciatic notches, unossified pubic bones
- Short, broad, and straight tubular bones with flared metaphyses
- Rounded, radiolucent appearance of proximal femoral end in most cases; squared proximal end with ragged metaphyseal margin in San Diego variant
- Very short and broad tubular bones of hands and feet

Mode of Inheritance: Autosomal dominant.

Molecular Basis: Specific Lys650Glu mutation of the *FGFR3* gene encoding the fibroblast growth factor receptor protein.

Prenatal Diagnosis: Ultrasound in the 2nd trimester can be confirmed by mutation analysis of *FGFR3* in cultured amniotic cells or cord blood cells.

Differential Diagnosis: *Thanatophoric dysplasia I* differs by the less frequent presence of a Kleeblattschädel and bowing of the long tubular bones, otherwise same differential diagnosis as thanatophoric dysplasia I.

Prognosis: No long-term survivors with this form of thanatophoric dysplasia have been reported.

Remarks: A mutation in the same FGFR3 codon as the thanatophoric dysplasia II mutation (Lys650Met) leads to severe achondroplasia with developmental delay and acanthosis nigricans (SADDAN) – but is compatible with survival into adulthood.

References

Chen CP, Chern SR, Shih JC, Wang W, Yeh LF, Chang TY, Tzen CY (2001) Prenatal diagnosis and genetic analysis of type I and type II thanatophoric dysplasia. Prenat Diagn 21:89–95

Langer LO, Yang SS, Hall JG, Sommer A, Kottamasu SR, Golabi M, Krassikoff N (1987) Thanatophoric dysplasia and cloverleaf skull. Am J Med Genet [Suppl] 3:167–179

Tavormina PL, Shiang R, Thompson LM, Zhu Y-Z, Wilkin DJ, Lachman RS, Wilcox WR, Rimoin DL, Cohn DH, Wasmuth JJ (1995) Thanatophoric dysplasia (types I and II) caused by distinct mutations in fibroblast growth factor receptor 3. Nature Genet 9: 321–328

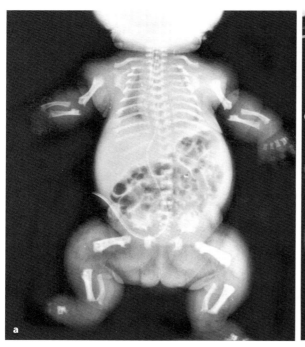
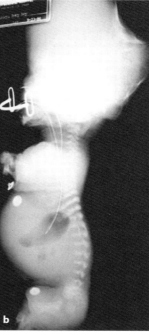

Fig. 3.3a, b. *Thanatophoric dysplasia II.* **a** The findings are similar to those in thanatophoric dysplasia I except for the femora which are straight. **b** The lateral view of the skull shows the upper and posterior bulge of the trilobar Kleeblattschädel. The vertebral bodies are not as severely flattened as in thanatophoric dysplasia I

Platyspondylic Dysplasia, Torrance-Luton Type   MIM 151210

Major Radiographic Features:
- Varying platyspondyly
- Hypoplasia of the lower ilial, short and broad ischial, and pubic bones
- Short and broad tubular bones with splayed and cupped metaphyses

Mode of Inheritance: Dominant.

Molecular Basis: Mutations in the C-propeptide region of the type II collagen gene (*COL2A1*).

Prenatal Diagnosis: Short limbs and retarded ossification of vertebral bodies by sonography.

Differential Diagnosis: In the *thanatophoric dysplasias* the tubular bones are more severely shortened. The femora are bowed in thanatophoric dysplasia I. Cranial abnormalities are common in thanatophoric dysplasia II, less frequent in thanatophoric dysplasia I, and have not been described in the Torrance-Luton type of platyspondylic dysplasia. *Achondroplasia* must be differentiated because of its good prognosis. It differs by the milder flattening of the vertebral bodies and the gland-like radiolucent aspect of the upper femoral ends.

Prognosis: Neonatal mortality is increased, but at least two females have survived into adulthood and gave birth to two affected children. Their adult height was 127 cm.

Remarks: The original description of the Torrance type of lethal platyspondylic dysplasias showed radiographic overlap with the San Diego type. Later observations showed milder manifestations. The spectrum of manifestations includes the milder Luton variant of lethal chondrodysplasias (Winter and Thompson 1982). Although the mortality is increased, it is not a lethal disease *sensu strictu.*

References

Horton WA, Rimoin DL, Hollister DW, Lachman RS (1979) Further heterogeneity within lethal neonatal short-limbed dwarfism: the platyspondylic types. J Pediatr 94:736–742

Kaibara N, Yokoyama K, Nakano H (1983) Torrance type of lethal neonatal short-limbed platyspondylic dwarfism. Skeletal Radiol 10: 17–19

Neumann L, Kunze J, Uhl M, Stöver B, Zabel B, Spranger J (2003) Survival to adulthood and dominant inheritance of platyspondylic skeletal dysplasia, Torrance-Luton type. Pediatr Radiol 33: 786–790

Nishimura G, Nakashima E, Mabuchi A et al (2004) Identification of COL2A1 mutations in platyspondylic skeletal dysplasia, Torrance type. J Med Genet 41:75–79

Omran H, Uhl M, Brandis M, Wolff G (2000) Survival and dominant transmission of "lethal" platyspondylic dwarfism of the "West coast" types. J Pediatr 136:411–413

Winter RM, Thompson EM (1982) Lethal, neonatal, short-limbed platyspondylic dwarfism. A further variant? Hum Genet 61:269–27

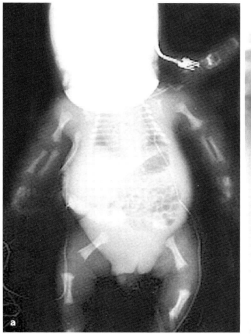
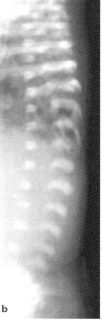

Fig. 3.4a, b. *Torrance-Luton Platyspondylic dysplasia.* Full-term newborn. **a** Major abnormalities are the small vertebral bodies, small ilia with horizontal acetabula and downward pointing spurs extending from their medial ends, short and broad tubular bones with slightly concave metaphyseal margins of the distal femora. **b** The vertebral bodies are insufficiently developed with small ossification centers in their anterior portions

Achondroplasia   MIM 100800

Synonyms: Chondrodystrophia fetalis, chondrodysplasia fetalis; chondrodystrophic dwarfism.

Major Radiographic Features:

- Large calvaria, short skull base, small occipital foramen
- Decrease of the interpedicular distance from upper to lower spine; short pedicles on lateral view
- Squared iliac bones with horizontal acetabular margins and small sacrosciatic notches
- Shortened tubular bones; oval radiolucent area in the proximal femur

Mode of Inheritance: Autosomal dominant; parental gonadal mosaicism observed to raise the recurrence risk of achondroplasia in sibs of unaffected parents to approximately 0.02%.

Molecular Basis: Point mutation at nucleotide 1138 of the cDNA of the *FGFR3* gene resulting in the substitution of an argine residue for a glycine in the fibroblast growth factor receptor 3.

Prenatal Diagnosis: Short femora have been detected after 20 weeks' gestation by ultrasound. A shortened base of the skull and depressed nasal bridge have also been detected. The specificity of short limbs is less than 0.25. Diagnostic ambiguity and errors are common. If one of the parents is affected, *FGFR3* can be determined in chorionic villi, fetal blood cells obtained by cordocentesis, or cultured fibroblasts from amniotic fluid.

Differential Diagnosis: The *thanatophoric dysplasias* and *homozygous achondroplasia* differ by the more severe flattening of the vertebral bodies and the more severe shortening of the tubular bones. The femora are bowed in thanatophoric dysplasia I, and cranial deformity due craniosynostosis is often present in thanatophoric dysplasia II. Another relatively common neonatal dysplasia with short limbs is *spondyloepiphyseal dysplasia congenita*. Ovoid vertebral bodies and absent ossification of the pubic bones characterize that dysplasia. Other neonatally manifest skeletal dysplasias are differentiated by characteristics described in the appropriate chapters.

Prognosis: Achondroplasia is not lethal. With proper care the patients survive the neonatal period and have a normal life expectancy.

Remarks: If both parents have achondroplasia, the risk of homozygous achondroplasia is 25%. Phenotypically it resembles thanatophoric dysplasia I. SADDAN dysplasia is a acronym for *severe achondroplasia with developmental delay and acanthosis nigricans*. This extremely rare disorder is caused by a lys650 met peculiar mutation at the nucleotide adjacent to the TD-II locus of the *FGFR3* gene (Bellus et al. 1999).

References

Bellus GA, Bamshad MJ, Przylepa KA, Dorst J, Lee RR, Hurko O, Jabs EW, Curry CJ, Wilcox WR, Lachman RS, Rimoin DL, Francomano CA (1999) Severe achondroplasia with developmental delay and acanthosis nigricans (SADDAN): phenotypic analysis of a new skeletal dysplasia caused by a Lys650Met mutation in fibroblast growth factor receptor 3. Am J Med Genet 85:53–65

Langer LO, Bauman PA, Gorlin J (1967) Achondroplasia. Am J Roentgenol 100:12–26

Mesoraca A, Pilu G, Perolo A et al (1996) Ultrasound and mid-trimester prenatal diagnosis of de novo achondroplasia. Prenat Diagn 16:764–768

Modaff P, Horton VK, Pauli RM (1996) Errors in the prenatal diagnosis of children with achondroplasia. Prenat Diagn 16:525–530

Spranger J, Brill PW, Poznanski A (2002) Bone Dysplasias. Urban and Fischer, Munich, pp 83–89

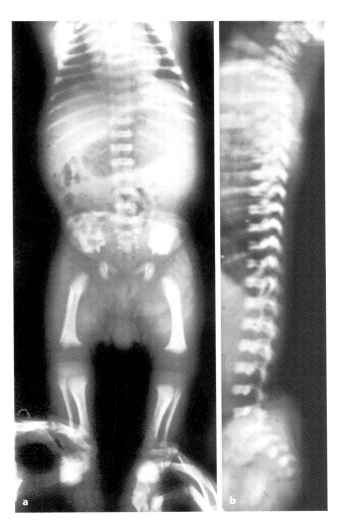

Fig. 3.5a, b. *Achondroplasia*, newborn. **a** The vertebral bodies are slightly flat. The interpedicular distances decrease from the upper to the lower lumbar spine. The ilia are squared with narrow sciatic notches and spurs extending downward from the medial ends of the horizontal acetabular roofs. The tubular bones are mildly shortened and curved. Note characteristic oval-shaped lucent appearance of the proximal femora.
b The vertebral bodies are slightly flat with remnants of coronal clefts appearing as central indentations of the upper and lower plates

Metatropic Dysplasia   MIM 156530, 250600

Synonym: Includes "Lethal metatropic dysplasia."

Major Radiographic Features:
- Small, flattened, often diamond-shaped vertebral bodies
- Narrow thorax
- Hypoplasia of the lower ilia with crescent-shaped iliac crests and low-set anteriosuperior iliac spines
- Shortened tubular bones with marked metaphyseal flare

Mode of Inheritance: Autosomal dominant; affected offspring of unaffected parents suggesting genetic heterogeneity or parental gonadal mosaicism.

Molecular Basis: Unknown.

Prenatal Diagnosis: Short limbs have been detected at 20 weeks' gestation.

Differential Diagnosis: Compared to lethal cases with metatropic dysplasia, the abnormalities in *fibrochondrogenesis* and *Schneckenbecken dysplasia* of the vertebrae, ilia and tubular bones are less severe. On the other hand, the bone changes in these two conditions are more severe than those in mildly affected patients with metatropic dysplasia.

Prognosis: The prognosis must be individually assessed on the basis of the bone changes. Infants with severely shortened and mushroomed tubular bones are stillborn or do not survive early infancy. Less severely affected infants may survive to adulthood and have children, but early mortality is increased due to respiratory failure secondary to craniocervical instability. Their intellectual development is normal.

Remarks: It is not clear if lethal and nonlethal metatropic dysplasia, as shown in the figures, are expressions of allelic mutations of the same gene or of nonallelic mutations of different genes. It has also been noted that metatropic dysplasia, fibrochondrogenesis, and Schneckenbecken dysplasia share a pattern of bone changes that may express a pathogenetic relationship.

References

Beck M, Roubicek M, Rogers JG, Naumoff P, Spranger J (1983) Heterogeneity of metatropic dysplasia. Eur J Pediatr 140: 231–237

Houston CS, Awen CF, Kent HP (1972) Fatal neonatal dwarfism. J Can Assoc Radiol 23 : 45–61

O'Sullivan MJ, McAllister WH, Ball RH, Teitelbaum SL, Swanson PE, Dehner LP (1998) Morphologic observations in a case of lethal variant (type I) metatropic dysplasia with atypical features: morphology of lethal metatropic dysplasia. Pediatr Dev Pathol 5: 405–412

Spranger JW, Brill PWE, Poznanski A (2002) Bone dysplasia, 2nd edn., Elsevier GmbH, Urban & Fischer, Munich

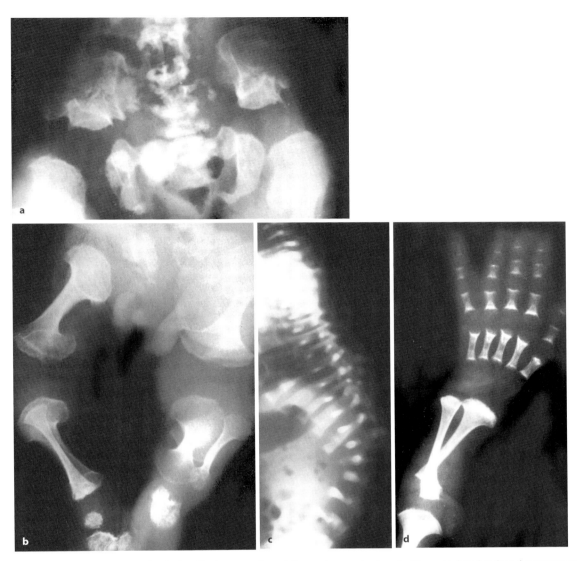

Fig. 3.6a–d. *Lethal metatropic dysplasia.* **a** The lower portions of the ilia are not developed and the anteriosuperior spines are deep set producing a halberd shape of the ilia. **b** The tubular bones are short and dumbbell shaped with very broad, mushroomed ends. **c** The vertebral bodies are underdeveloped, more severely in their dorsal than in their anterior portions, giving them a teardrop shape. **d** Radius and ulna are shortened with grossly flared ends and convex metaphyseal margins. The ends of the short tubular bones are slightly wide with scalloped proximal and distal margins. (From: Spranger et al.: Bone Dysplasias, 2nd edn., 2002, with kind permission from Elsevier GmbH, Urban & Fischer, Munich)

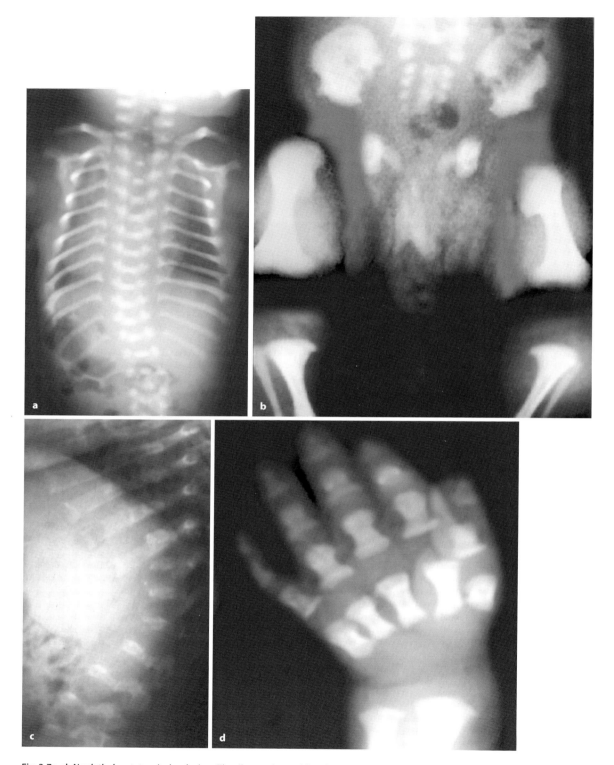

Fig. 3.7a–d. *Nonlethal metatropic dysplasia.* **a** The ribs are short with splayed ends. The vertebral bodies are flat. **b** The basilar portions of the ilia are slightly hypoplastic. The femora are short with broad, hyperplastic ends. **c** Flattened vertebral bodies and wide intervertebral spaces are seen. **d** Metacarpals and phalanges are short and dumbbell shaped

Fibrochondrogenesis   MIM 228520

Major Radiographic Features:

- Defective ossification of the posterior parts of the vertebral bodies
- Short ribs with splayed ends
- Small ilia with spurs extending caudally from the acetabular roof
- Short tubular bones with bulbous ends

Mode of Inheritance: Autosomal recessive.

Molecular Basis: Unknown.

Prenatal Diagnosis: Short limbs and deficient ossification of the vertebral bodies may be detected by ultrasound in the 2nd trimester.

Differential Diagnosis: *Schneckenbecken dysplasia* is radiologically similar and may be etiopathogenetically related. The tubular shortening is usually less severe in Schneckenbecken dysplasia. The skeletal abnormalities in lethal metatropic dysplasia are also similar, but more severe than in fibrochondrogenesis.

Prognosis: All reported patients died at or soon after birth.

References

Hunt NCA, Vujanic GM (1998) Fibrochondrogenesis in a 17-week fetus: a case expanding the phenotype. Am J Med Genet 75: 326–329

Lazzaroni-Fossati F, Stanescu V, Stanescu R, Serra G, Magliano P, Maroteaux P (1978) La fibrochondrogénèse. Arch Fr Pédiatr 35: 1096–1104

Whitley CM, Langer LO, Ophoven J, Gilbert EF, Gonzalez C, Mammel M, Coleman M, Rosemberg S, Rodriques CJ, Sibley R, Horton WA, Opitz JM, Gorlin JR (1984) Fibrochondrogenesis: lethal, autosomal recessive chondrodysplasia with distinctive cartilage histopathology. Am J Med Genet 19:265–275

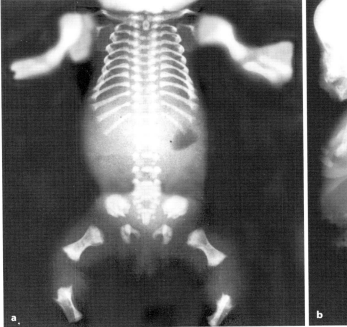
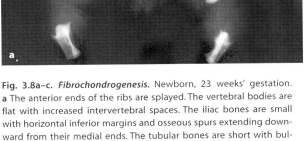
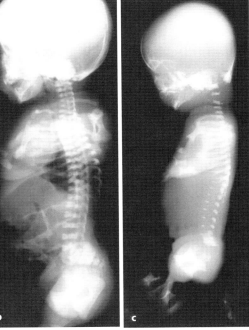

Fig. 3.8a–c. *Fibrochondrogenesis.* Newborn, 23 weeks' gestation. a The anterior ends of the ribs are splayed. The vertebral bodies are flat with increased intervertebral spaces. The iliac bones are small with horizontal inferior margins and osseous spurs extending downward from their medial ends. The tubular bones are short with bulbous ends. b Coronal clefts separate diamond-shaped anterior portions of the vertebral bodies from small dorsal ossification centers. c In this 23 week old fetus ossification of the vertebral bodies is reduced to thin, wafer-like structures. The cervical and upper thoracic vertebral bodies are not ossified at all

Schneckenbecken Dysplasia   MIM 269250

Major Radiographic Features:

- Hypoplastic vertebral bodies
- Short ribs with splayed ends
- Small ilia with medial projection from the inner margins (snail-like appearance)
- Shortened, dumbbell-shaped tubular bones

Mode of Inheritance: Autosomal recessive.

Molecular Basis: Unknown.

Prenatal Diagnosis: Short limbs were detected by ultrasound at 16 weeks' gestation.

Differential Diagnosis: Compared to *fibrochondrogenesis* the medial protrusion of the ilia is more pronounced and the ends of the tubular bones are less bulbous in Schneckenbecken dysplasia. In *lethal metatropic* dysplasia the ends of the tubular bones are more severely expanded with convex joint surfaces.

Prognosis: All reported patients were stillborn or died shortly after birth.

References

Borochowitz Z, Jones KL, Silbey R, Adomian G, Lachman R, Rimoin DL (1986) A distinct lethal neonatal chondrodysplasia with snail-like pelvis: Schneckenbecken dysplasia. Am J Med Genet 25:46–59

Nikkels PG, Stigter RH, Knol IE, van der Harten JH (2001) Schneckenbecken dysplasia, radiology and histology. Pediatr Radiol 31:27/30

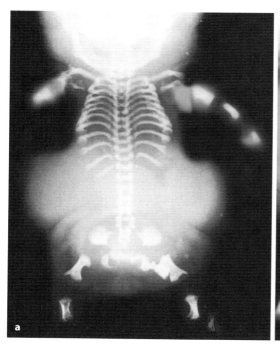
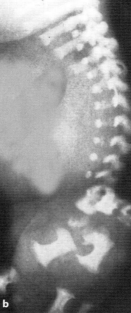

Fig. 3.9a, b. *Schneckenbecken dysplasia.*
a Stillborn. The ribs are short with splayed anterior ends. The vertebral bodies are small. The iliac bones are small, round, with a medial osseous projection producing a snail-like configuration. The tubular bones are short and dumbbell shaped with slightly convex margins of the proximal femora and irregular metaphyseal margins of the distal femora and proximal humeri.
b Newborn, 34 weeks' gestation. Small, round ossification centers are seen in the anterior portions of the vertebral bodies. Both infants are hydropic

Lethal Metaphyseal Chondrodysplasia, Sedaghatian Type   MIM 250220

Synonym: Lethal metaphyseal chondrodysplasia, Shiraz type.

Major Radiographic Features:
- Small thorax
- Mild platyspondyly
- Flat and broad iliac wings
- Shortened tubular bones with metaphyseal cupping and irregularity

Mode of Inheritance: Autosomal recessive.

Molecular Basis: Unknown.

Prenatal Diagnosis: Short limbs have been detected by ultrasound at 31 weeks' gestation.

Differential Diagnosis: *Thanatophoric dysplasia* and *other lethal chondrodysplasias* differ by more severe flattening of the vertebral bodies and more severe shortening of the tubular bones. In *hypochondrogenesis* and *spondyloepiphyseal dysplasia congenita* the pubic bones are characteristically unossified. *Jansen metaphyseal dysplasia* is differentiated by the associated undermineralization.

Prognosis: Most patients are stillborn or die within the first days of life of cardiorespiratory failure. A single patient has been kept alive with respiratory assistance for 161 days.

Remarks: Myocardial necrosis, porencephaly, and lissencephaly have been described in some patients.

References
Elcioglu N, Hall CM (1998) Spondylometaphyseal dysplasia – Sedaghatian type. Am J Med Genet 76:410–414

Sedaghatian MR (1980) Congenital lethal metaphyseal chondrodysplasia: a newly recognized complex autosomal recessive disorder. Am J Med Genet 6:269–274

Opitz JM, Spranger JW, Stöss HR, Pesch HJ, Azadeh B (1987) Sedaghatian congenital lethal metaphyseal chondrodysplasia – observations in a second Iranian family and histopathological studies. Am J Med Genet 26:583–590

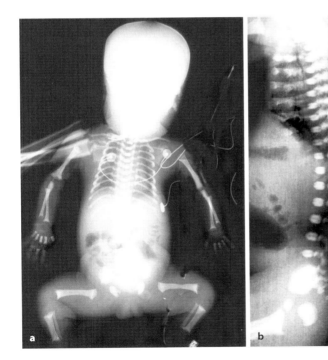
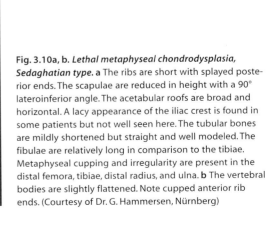

Fig. 3.10a, b. *Lethal metaphyseal chondrodysplasia, Sedaghatian type.* **a** The ribs are short with splayed posterior ends. The scapulae are reduced in height with a 90° lateroinferior angle. The acetabular roofs are broad and horizontal. A lacy appearance of the iliac crest is found in some patients but not well seen here. The tubular bones are mildly shortened but straight and well modeled. The fibulae are relatively long in comparison to the tibiae. Metaphyseal cupping and irregularity are present in the distal femora, tibiae, distal radius, and ulna. **b** The vertebral bodies are slightly flattened. Note cupped anterior rib ends. (Courtesy of Dr. G. Hammersen, Nürnberg)

Achondrogenesis 1A   MIM 200600

Synonym: Houston-Harris type of Achondrogenesis.

Major Radiographic Features:
- Poorly ossified skull
- Unossified vertebral bodies
- Short ribs with multiple fractures
- Hypoplastic ilia with horizontal, arched lower margins
- Short, misshapen, often stellate tubular bones with minimal tubulation

Mode of Inheritance: Autosomal recessive.

Molecular Basis: Unknown.

Prenatal Diagnosis: In the second trimester short limbs are detectable by ultrasound. Hydramnios and hydrops may be found.

Differential Diagnosis: In *achondrogenesis IB* there are no rib fractures and tubulation of the long bones is completely absent. *Achondrogenesis II* differs by the retained longitudinal axis of the tubular bones and better ossified vertebral bodies. *Hypophosphatasia* does not show the stellate, globular appearance of the tubular bones.

Prognosis: All known patients have been stillborn or died shortly after birth.

Reference

Borochowitz Z, Lachman R, Adomian GE, Spear G, Jones K, Rimoin DL (1988) Achondrogenesis type I: delineation of further heterogeneity and identification of two distinct subgroups. J Pediatr 112: 23–31

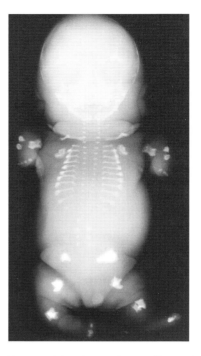

Fig. 3.11. *Achondrogenesis I-A.* Stillborn infant, 30 weeks' gestation. The calvaria is insufficiently ossified. The ribs are short with splayed ends. Slightly irregular contours in the left 6th and 7th ribs are compatible with multiple fractures that are frequently found in this condition. Vertebral bodies and ischial and pubic bones are not ossified. The lower ilia are not developed. The tubular bones are strikingly short, with concave ends, sometimes accentuated by longitudinal spurs extending from their ends. Radius and ulna are seen as small, round bone islands. Ossification of the short tubular bones is severely deficient

Achondrogenesis 1B   MIM 600972

Synonym: Achondrogenesis, Fraccaro-(Parenti) type.

Major Radiographic Features:

- Poorly ossified calvaria
- Unossified vertebral bodies
- Short ribs without fractures
- Small ilia with concave medial and inferior margins; unossified pubic and ischial bones
- Globular or stellate long tubular bones lacking axial alignment

Mode of Inheritance: Autosomal recessive.

Molecular Basis: Mutations in the *DTDST* gene encoding the cellular sulfate transporter; allelic mutations causing atelosteogenesis type II, diastrophic dysplasia, and autosomal recessive epiphyseal dysplasia.

Prenatal Diagnosis: Sonographic recognition is possible in the second trimester on the basis of short limbs, reduced echogenicity of spine and head, narrow thorax, protuberant abdomen, hydramnios. If the mutation is known from a previously affected sibling, mutational analysis of the *DTDST* gene is possible in fetal cells.

Differential Diagnosis: In *achondrogenesis 1A* longitudinal orientation of the tubular bones is partially preserved and the ribs show multiple fractures. *Achondrogenesis 2* differs by the short, but tubulated long bones and the better ossification of the vertebral bodies. *Atelosteogenesis II* shows better ossification of the vertebrae and longitudinally oriented tubular bones. *Hypophosphatasia* is differentiated by the severe but erratic ossification defects and preserved longitudinal orientation of ossified portions of the tubular bones.

Prognosis: Death occurs in utero or within hours after birth.

Remarks: Achondrogenesis 1B is one of a family of bone dysplasias caused by mutations of the *DTDST* gene. Others members are de la Chapelle dysplasia, diastrophic dysplasia, and autosomal recessive multiple epiphyseal dysplasia. Varying phenotypes are caused by different degrees of residual activity of the sulfate transporter protein.

References

Borochowitz Z, Lachman R, Adomian GE, Spear G, Jones K, Rimoin DL (1988) Achondrogenesis type I: delineation of further heterogeneity and identification of two distinct subgroups. J Pediatr 112: 23–31

Rossi A, Superti-Furga A (2001) Mutations in the diastrophic dysplasia sulfate transporter (DTDST) gene (SLC26A2): 22 novel mutations, mutation review, associated skeletal phenotypes, and diagnostic relevance. Hum Mutat 17:159–171

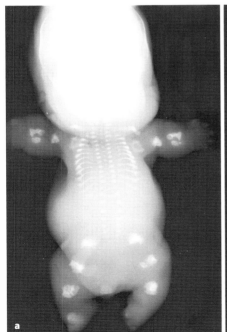
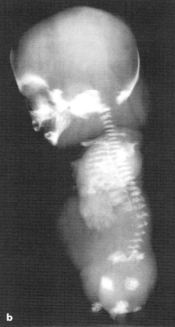

Fig. 3.12a, b. *Achondrogenesis 1B*, 30-weeks' gestation. The calvaria is poorly ossified. The ribs are short with splayed anterior ends. The scapulae are misshapen. Thin, wafer-like ossification centers are seen in some vertebral bodies of the thoracic spine; the pedicles are well ossified. Only the superior portions of the ilia are mineralized; pubic and ischial bones are not ossified. The long bones are not tubulated and appear as stellate, ragged, or nondescript structures

Achondrogenesis Type 2/Hypochondrogenesis   MIM 200610

Synonym: Achondrogenesis, Langer-Saldino type.

Major Radiographic Features:

- Absent ossification of the cervical vertebral bodies, severely retarded ossification of the vertebral bodies of the thoracic and lumbar spine; absent ossification of the sacrum
- Barrel-shaped thorax with short ribs
- Small iliac bones with crescent-shaped inner and inferior margins; absent or severely delayed ossification of the pubic and ischial bones
- Very short tubular bones with metaphyseal flare and cupping

Mode of Inheritance: Autosomal dominant.

Molecular Basis: Mutations of the *COL2A1* gene encoding type II collagen molecules.

Prenatal Diagnosis: Short limbs and frequently hydrops are recognized by ultrasound in the second trimester of pregnancy. If the mutation is known from an affected parent, mutation analysis of the *COL2A1* gene can be performed in fetal cells.

Differential Diagnosis: In *achondrogenesis 1A* the ribs are thinner, with evidence of multiple fractures; the vertebral bodies are not ossified; and the tubular bones are more severely shortened and misshapen. In *achondrogenesis 1B* the vertebral bodies are not ossified and the tubular bones are not longitudinally oriented. *Kniest dysplasia* and *spondyloepiphyseal dysplasia congenita* show slightly better ossification of the vertebral bodies and pelvic bones, and the long bones are better tubulated and not as short.

Prognosis: Affected individuals are usually delivered prematurely. Patients with achondrogenesis II are stillborn or die within a few hours. Children with hypochondrogenesis are usually born alive and may survive with the aid of supportive measures. Depending on the intensity of life support they die within the first days to months from cardiorespiratory failure.

Remarks: Achondrogenesis II, hypochondrogenesis, Kniest dysplasia, and spondyloepiphyseal dysplasia are caused by allelic mutations of the same gene encoding type 2 collagen. Although phenotypically and prognostically they form a continuous spectrum, the nosologic distinction of different entities within the type 2 collagenopathies is justified because of their different prognosis.

References

Borochowitz Z, Ornoy A, Lachman R, Rimoin DL (1986) Achondrogenesis II – hypochondrogenesis: variability versus heterogeneity. Am J Med Genet 24:273–288

Spranger J, Winterpacht A, Zabel B (1994) The type II collagenopathies: a spectrum of chondrodysplasias. Eur J Pediatr 153:56–65

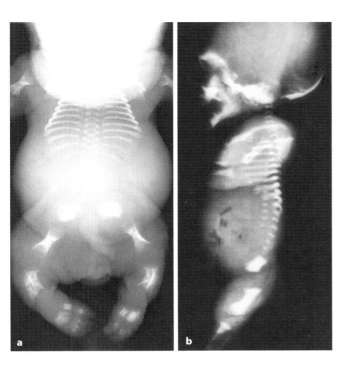

Fig. 3.13a, b. *Achondrogenesis 2.* **a** The ribs are short and horizontally oriented. Except for the bodies of the thoracic vertebrae and the neural arches of the lower cervical, thoracic, and upper lumbar spine, the spine is not ossified. There is no ossification of the sacrum or pubic and ischial bones. The ilia are vertically short with concave lower and medial borders. The tubular bones are short and broad with concave metaphyseal margins. **b** Note short ribs and deficient ossification of the vertebrae in the cervical and lumbar spine

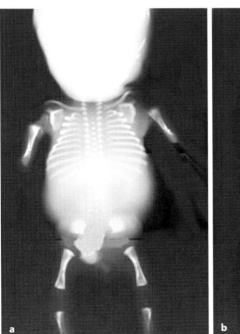
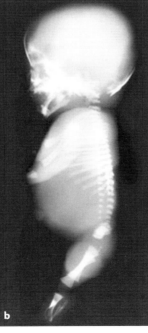

Fig. 3.14a, b. *Hypochondrogenesis*, 38 weeks' gestation. The chest is small and broad. Ossification of the truncal skeleton is severely retarded with small ossification centers in the thoracic and lumbar vertebral bodies, but no ossification of the cervical vertebral bodies, sacrum, pubic bones, ischial bones, and lower portions of the ilia. The long tubular bones are shortened but well modeled

Kniest Dysplasia/Spondyloepiphyseal Dysplasia Congenita   MIM 156550/183900

Synonym: SED congenita.

Major Radiographic Features:

- Flattened, ovoid vertebral bodies, sometimes with coronal clefts
- Small ilia due to hypoplasia of the inferior portions
- Absent ossification of the pubic bones
- Shortened tubular bones; more severe in Kniest dysplasia than in SED congenita
- Dumbbell-shaped femora in Kniest dysplasia

Mode of Inheritance: Autosomal dominant.

Molecular Basis: Mutations of the gene encoding type 2 collagen (*Col2A1*); single base mutations, deletion, or duplication of part the gene cause SED congenita; in-frame deletions or exon skipping lead to the Kniest phenotype.

Prenatal Diagnosis: Short limbs are detected by sonography. If the mutation is known from an affected parent, mutation analysis of the *COL2A1* gene is possible in chorionic villi or amnion cells.

Differential Diagnosis: In achondrogenesis 2 and hypochondrogenesis, ossification of the spine and pelvis is more severely retarded and the tubular bones are more severely shortened.

Prognosis: In contrast to newborns with achondrogenesis 2 or hypochondrogenesis, survival chances of patients with SED congenita and of most patients with Kniest dysplasia are good.

Remarks: Mutations of the *COL11A2* gene encoding a strand of the trimeric type 11 collagen cause otospondylomegaepiphyseal dysplasia (OSMED) which in the neonate is almost indistinguishable from Kniest dysplasia. Differentiation of the two disorders requires molecular analysis. The nosology of the type 2 collagenopathies is discussed in the chapter on achondrogenesis 2/hypochondrogenesis.

References

Spranger J, Winterpacht A, Zabel B (1994) The type II collagenopathies: a spectrum of chondrodysplasias. Eur J Pediatr 153 : 56–65

Weis MA, Wilkin DJ, Kim HJ, Wilcox WR, Lachman RS, Rimoin DL, Cohn DH, Eyre DR (1998) Structurally abnormal type II collagen in a severe form of Kniest dysplasia caused by an exon 24 skipping mutation. J Biol Chem 273 : 4761– 4768

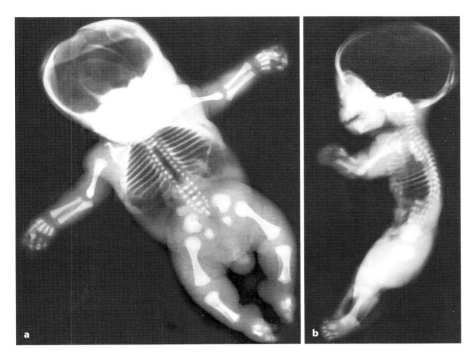

Fig. 3.15a, b. *Kniest dysplasia.* Stillborn **a** The thorax is short and broad. The lumbar vertebral bodies are flat; the thoracic vertebrae have been removed at autopsy. The pubic bones are not ossified, the ischial bones are short and broad. The tubular bones are short with flared ends. **b** Note coronal clefts of the vertebral bodies. The cervical bodies are not ossified

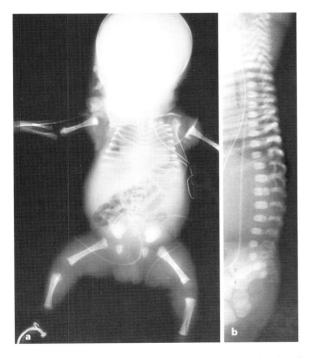

Fig. 3.16a, b. *Spondyloepiphyseal dysplasia congenita.* The chest is small, the vertebral bodies are flat and ovoid. A coronal cleft is seen in L2. There is no ossification of the pubic bones and the tubular bones are shorter than normal. These changes are similar to those in hypochondrogenesis (Fig. 3.14) but less severe

Dyssegmental Dysplasia   MIM 224400

Includes Silverman-Handmaker type, Rolland-Desbuquois type.

Major Radiographic Features:
- Irregularly sized and formed vertebral bodies with single or multiple ossification centers, more severe in the Silverman-Handmaker than in the Rolland-Desbuquois phenotype
- Small iliac bones; short and thick pubic and ischial bones
- Shortened, wide, often angulated long tubular bones

Mode of Inheritance: Autosomal recessive.

Molecular Basis: Severe cases with the Silverman-Handmaker phenotype are the expression of a null mutation of the perlecan gene *HSPG2* located on chromosome 1p36.1.-35. Cases with the Rolland-Desbuquois phenotype may be allelic variants.

Prenatal Diagnosis: Short, bowed limbs and grossly disorganized vertebral bodies have been recognized at 20 weeks' gestation.

Differential Diagnosis: The skeletal abnormalities in the *Schwartz-Jampel syndrome* are similar but less severe than in dyssegmental dysplasia. Other forms of *congenital bowing of the long bones* are not associated with vertebral segmentation defects.

Prognosis: The prognosis varies with the severity of the bone lesions. Severely affected newborns with the Silverman-Handmaker phenotype are stillborn or die within the first days of life. A single patient has been reported who survived to 8 months of age with marked mental deficiency, defective hearing, and unexplained episodes of hyperthermia. Patients with the less severe Rolland-Desbuquois phenotype may survive to childhood and possibly later.

Remarks: Phenotypically, the Silverman-Handmaker and the Rolland-Desbuquois phenotypes are part of a continuous spectrum and may be allelic variants. However, genetic heterogeneity has not been excluded.

References

Aleck KA, Grix A, Clericuzio C, Kaplan P, Adomian GE, Lachman R, Rimoin DL (1987) Dyssegmental dysplasias: clinical, radiographic and morphologic evidence of heterogeneity. Am J Med Genet 27:295–312

Andersen PE, Hauge M, Bang J (1988) Dyssegmental dysplasia in siblings: prenatal ultrasonic diagnosis. Skeletal Radiol 17:29–31

Arikawa-Hirasawa E, Wilcox WR, Yamada Y (2001) Dyssegmental dysplasia, Silverman-Handmaker type: unexpected role of perlecan in cartilage development. Am J Med Genet 106:254–257

D'Orey MC, Mateus M, Guimaraes H, Miguel C, Costeira MJ, Nogueira R, Montenegro N, Santos NT, Maroteaux P (1997) Dyssegmental dysplasia: a case report of a Rolland-Desbuquois type. Pediatr Radiol 27:9489–950

Prabhu VG, Kozma C, Leftridge CA, Helmbrecht GD, France ML (1998) Dyssegmental dysplasia Silverman-Handmaker type in a consanguineous Druze Lebanese family: long term survival and documentation of the natural history. Am J Med Genet 13:7164–7170

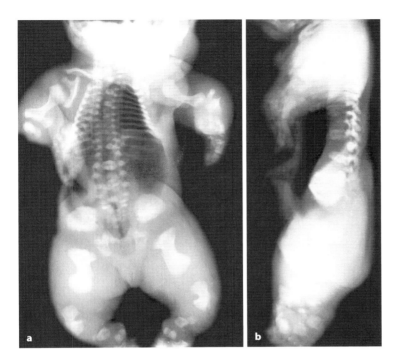

Fig. 3.17a, b. *Dyssegmental dysplasia, Silverman-Handmaker type.* The vertebral bodies vary in size and shape. Multiple ossification centers are seen in some; other vertebral bodies are not ossified at all. The lower portions of the ilia are not developed; the pubic and ischial bones are broad. The long tubular bones are short and bowed with wide ends

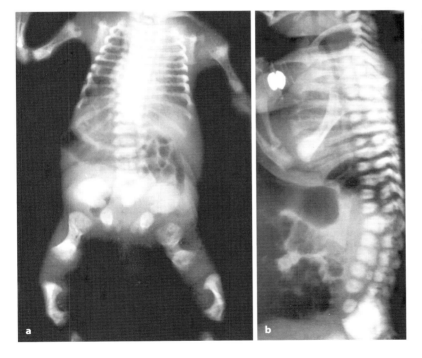

Fig. 3.18a, b. *Dyssegmental dysplasia, Rolland-Desbuquois type.* The bone changes in this patient are similar but less severe than in the Silverman-Handmaker type (Fig. 3.17). Characteristics seen in both phenotypes are the irregular size and shape of the vertebral bodies, small ilia with wide pubic and ischial bones, and the distorted dumbbell shape of the femora. In other patients, femoral and tibial bowing may be less pronounced

Schwartz-Jampel Syndrome   MIM 255800

Synonym: Myotonic chondrodysplasia, Catel-Hempel syndrome.

Major Radiographic Features:

- Mildly flattened vertebral bodies; coronal clefts
- Flared iliac wings with supra-acetabular lateral notches and wide ischial bones
- Short and bowed femora and tibiae with wide ends

Mode of Inheritance: Autosomal recessive.

Molecular Basis: Mutations of the gene encoding perlecan (*HSPG2*) on chromosome 1p34-p36.1

Prenatal Diagnosis: Short and bowed femora may be detected by ultrasound.

Differential Diagnosis: *Kniest dysplasia* may present with coronal clefts of the vertebral bodies and short femora but differs by the retarded ossification of the pubic bones, absence of the supra-acetabular notch, and absence of femoral bowing. Grossly irregular ossification of the vertebral bodies is seen in *dyssegmental dysplasia* but not in the Schwartz-Jampel syndrome.

Prognosis: In severely affected infants early feeding and respiratory difficulties have been reported and their prognosis is guarded. Prolonged ventilatory assistance may be needed. Myotonia usually manifests in childhood. Bowing of the long bones (kyphomelia) may persist to an older age and some of the affected children have been misdiagnosed as "kyphomelic dysplasia."

Remarks: Dyssegmental dysplasia and Schwartz-Jampel syndrome are part of a continuous spectrum of clinical disorders caused by allelic mutations of the perlecan gene.

References

Al Gazali LI, Varghese M, Varady E, Al Talabani J, Scorer J, Bakalinova D (1996) Neonatal Schwartz-Jampel syndrome: a common autosomal recessive syndrome in the United Arab Emirates. J Med Genet 33:203–211

Arikawa-Hirasama E, Le AH, Nishino I, Nonaka I, Ho NC, Francomano CA, Govindraj P, Hassel J, Devaney JM, Spranger J, Stevenson RE, Iannaccone S, Dalakas MC, Yamada Y (2002) Structural and functional mutations of the perlecan gene cause Schwartz-Jampel syndrome, with myotonic myopathy and chondrodysplasia. Am J Hum Genet 70:1368–1375

Spranger J, Hall BD, Hane B, Srivasta A, Stevenson RE (2000) The spectrum of Schwartz-Jampel syndrome includes micromelic chondrodysplasia, kyphomelic dysplasia, and Burton disease. Am J Med Genet 94:287–295

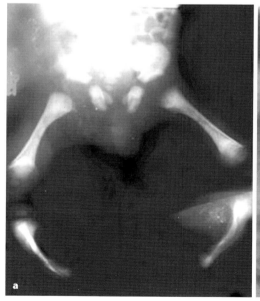
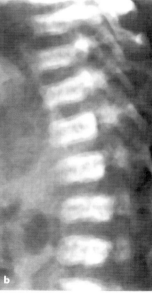

Fig. 3.19a, b. *Schwartz-Jampel syndrome.* Full-term newborn. **a** The iliac bodies are hypoplastic. A lateral supra-acetabular notch is best seen on the right side. The tubular bones are short with wide ends. There is mild bowing of the femora and distinct bowing of the tibiae. **b** The thoracic vertebral bodies are slightly flat. Remnants of coronal clefts are seen in the lower bodies

Cartilage-Hair Hypoplasia   MIM 250250

Synonym: Metaphyseal chondrodysplasia, McKusick type; Round femoral, inferior epiphysis dysplasia.

Major Radiographic Features:
- Shortened long tubular bones
- Curved femora, occasionally with well ossified, round distal femoral epiphyses
- Sometimes short ribs and anterior angulation of the sternum

Mode of Inheritance: Autosomal recessive.

Molecular Basis: Mutations of the *RMRP* gene located on 9p13 encoding the RNA component of a ribonucleo-protein endoribonuclease.

Prenatal Diagnosis: In late pregnancy short and bowed femora may be detected by ultrasound. If the mutation is known from a sibling, molecular analysis of the *RMRP* gene can be attempted.

Differential Diagnosis: *Campomelic dysplasia* differs by hypoplastic scapulae, hypoplastic thoracic vertebral pedicles, and narrow iliac bones. Radio-humeral synostosis and craniosynostosis are present in the *Antley-Bixler* syndrome but not in cartilage-hair hypoplasia. The *Schwartz-Jampel syndrome* is differentiated by the presence of vertebral anomalies. Bone density and bone thickness are normal in cartilage-hair hypoplasia and decreased in other forms of *congenital bowing* of the femora.

Prognosis: Neonatal and early development is usually normal. Later complications include impaired immunity, Hirschsprung disease, and a higher rate of malignancy. Adult height ranges between 111 cm and 151 cm in males, and between 104 cm and 137 cm in females.

Remarks: Some patients with persistent bowing of the femora have been misnamed "kyphomelic dysplasia." Cases with prominent, round distal femoral epiphyses have been called "Glasgow variant."

References

Mäkitie O, Marttinen E, Kaitila I (1992) Skeletal growth in cartilage-hair hypoplasia. Pediatr Radiol 22:434–439

Mäkitie O, Kaitila I, Savilahti E (1998) Susceptibility to infections and in vitro immune functions in cartilage-hair hypoplasia. Eur J Pediatr 157:816–820

Corder WT, Hummel M, Miller C, Wilson NW (1995) Association of kyphomelic dysplasia with severe combined immunodeficiency. Am J Med Genet 17:616–619

Lecora M, Parenti G, Iaccarino E, Scarano G, Cucchiara S, Andria G (1995) Immunological disorder and Hirschsprung disease in round femoral inferior epiphysis dysplasia. Clin Dysmorphol 4:130–135

Sulisalo T, Sillence D, Wilson M, Rzzanen M, Kaitila I (1995) Early prenatal diagnosis of cartilage-hair hypoplasia (CHH) with polymorphic DNA markers. Prenat Diagn 15:135–140

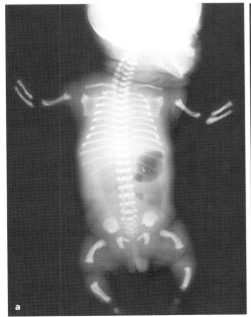
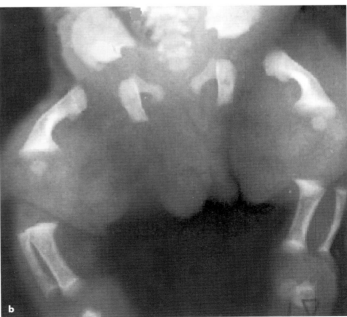

Fig. 3.20a, b. *Cartilage-hair hypoplasia*. a The iliac bones are short and round due to hypoplasia of the iliac bodies. The tubular bones are short with bowing of the femora and, less conspicuously, the other long bones. **b** Large, round distal femoral epiphyses are seen in this full-term newborn

Campomelic Dysplasia   MIM 211990, 114290

Synonym: Campomelic syndrome, which includes acampomelic campomelic dysplasia.

Major Radiographic Features:

- Hypoplastic scapulae
- Small, bell-shaped chest with eleven pairs of ribs
- Abnormal cervical vertebrae
- Nonmineralized vertebrae
- Vertical, narrow iliac wings; widely spaced vertical ischia; hypoplastic pubic bones
- Dislocated hips
- Bowed femora and tibiae
- Hypoplastic fibulae
- Dislocated radial heads
- Short first metacarpals; short middle phalanges of 2nd through 5th fingers

Mode of Inheritance: Autosomal dominant.

Molecular Basis: Mutations of the *SOX9* gene on chromosome 17p24.3-q25.1 or chromosomal rearrangements outside the coding region; *SOX9* encoded protein acts as transcription factor regulating chondrogenesis via *COL2A1* and sex determination via *SRY* in early embryogenesis.

Prenatal Diagnosis: Shortened and/or bowed femora and tibiae have been detected at 17 weeks' gestation. This finding is nonspecific and, in addition to campomelic dysplasia, occurs in osteogenesis imperfecta, hypophosphatasia, dyssegmental dysplasia, Schwartz-Jampel syndrome, Antley-Bixler syndrome, and others. Straight femora do not rule out campomelic syndrome. Hypoplastic scapulae are more specific for campomelic dysplasia.

Differential Diagnosis: Undermineralized bone structure differentiates disorders with congenital osteopenia such as *osteogenesis imperfecta*, *hypophosphatasia*, *Stüve-Wiedemann syndrom*e. *Intrauterine hypomobility* with or without *arthrogryposis* is associated with thin, slender bone shafts. Craniosynostosis and humeroradial synostosis characterize the *Antley-Bixler syndrome*. Other disorders with *congenital bowing* and normal bone density do not exhibit the hypoplastic scapulae and vertebrae characterizing campomelic dysplasia.

Prognosis: Infantile mortality is increased due to cardiorespiratory insufficiency. Survivors may develop progressive kyphoscoliosis. Mild tibial bowing, hypoplastic scapulae and fibulae have been observed in the mother of a severely affected child with campomelic dysplasia (Lynch et al. 1993). Some survivors have been mentally retarded. Patients with a chromosomal rearrangement involving 17q23.3-q25.1 have often a milder phenotype. The degree of femoral bowing is not related to the outcome. Renal anomalies and absent olfactory bulbs and tracts have been found at autopsy.

Remarks: Defective expression of *SRY* causes sex reversal or ambiguous genitalia in approximately three-quarters of chromosomal males with campomelic dysplasia.

References

Houston CS, Opitz JM, Spranger JW, Macpherson RI, Reed MH Gilbert EF, Herrmann J, Schinzel A (1983) The campomelic syndrome: report of 17 cases, and follow-up on the currently 17-year old boy first reported by Maroteaux et al in 1971. Am J Med Genet 15:3–28

Lynch SA, Gaunt ML, Minford AMB (1993) Campomelic dysplasia: evidence of autosomal dominant inheritance. J Med Genet 30: 638–686

Mansour S, Hall CM, Pembrey ME, Young ID (1995) A clinical and genetic study of campomelic dysplasia. J Med Genet 32: 415–420

Meyer J, Sudbeck P, Held M et al (1997) Mutational analysis of the SOX9 gene in campomelic dysplasia and autosomal sex reversal: lack of genotype/phenotype correlations. Hum Mol Genet 6: 91–98

Sanders RC, Greyson-Fleg RT, Hogge WA, Blakemore KJ, McGowan KD, Isbister S (1994) Osteogenesis imperfecta and campomelic dysplasia: difficulties in prenatal diagnosis. J Ultrasound Med 13: 691–700

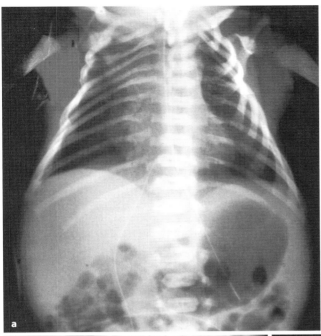

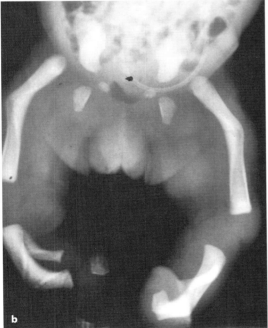

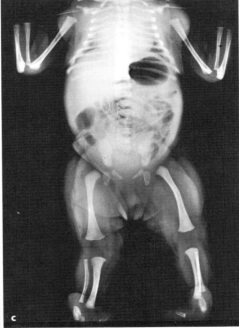

Fig. 3.21a–c. *Campomelic dysplasia.* **a** The thoracic inlet is small and the chest bell shaped. Ossification of the ribs is irregular. There are 11 pairs of ribs. A small scapula is seen on the left side, but not on the right. The thoracic vertebral pedicles are not seen. **b** The iliac wings are narrow, the acetabula poorly ossified, the pubic bones small, and the hips dislocated. The femora, tibiae, and fibulae are short and bowed; the fibulae are hypoplastic. **c** *Acampomelic campomelic dysplasia.* The bone changes are similar to those in **a** and **b** except for the long bones which are not or only slightly bowed

Antley-Bixler Syndrome   MIM 207410

Synonym: Multiple synostotic osteodysgenesis, acrocephalosynankie.

Major Radiographic Features:
- Femoral bowing
- Humeroradial synostosis
- Neonatal fractures
- Hypoplastic scapulae
- Craniosynostosis

Mode of Inheritance: Heterogeneous; autosomal dominant, autosomal recessive, intrauterine exposure to fluconazole; overall female/male ratio 3/1.

Molecular Basis: Heterozygous mutations of fibroblast growth factor receptor 2 in some cases, unknown in others.

Prenatal Diagnosis: Bowing of long bones, immobility at the elbows, humeroradial synostosis have been detected by ultrasound in the 17th week of gestation.

Differential Diagnosis: *Campomelic dysplasia* differs by the presence of hypoplastic thoracic pedicles and cervical vertebrae and by the absence of neonatal fractures, radiohumeral synostosis, and craniosynostosis. Differentiation of the two conditions may difficult and require molecular analysis of *SOX*9. Hypoplastic scapulae are found in both conditions but not in *other bowing syndromes*. For further differentiation see campomelic dysplasia.

Prognosis: Neonatal mortality is increased, mostly due to respiratory insufficiency associated with choanal stenosis. With intensive medical care, the patients may survive and grow up with normal intellectual development.

Remarks: Clinical manifestations of the Antley-Bixler syndrome include hypoplastic labia, enlarged clitoris and other genital abnormalities associated with abnormal steroid profiles. These latter are present in approximately half of the female patients pointing to the heterogeneity of the disorder, which represents a phenotype rather than a causally defined syndrome. The teratogenic effect of fluconazole has only been observed with doses above 400 mg/day that may have induced a disordered steroidogenesis (Reardon et al. 2000).

References

Aleck KA, Bartley DL (1997) Multiple malformation syndrome following fluconazole use in pregnancy: report of an additional patients. Am J Med Genet 72:253–256

Crisponi G, Porcu C, Piu ME (1997) Antley-Bixler syndrome: case report and review of the literature. Clin Dysmorphol 6:61–68

Escobar LF Bixler D, Sadove M, Bull MJ (1988) Antley-Bixler syndrome from a prognostic perspective: report of a case and review of the literature. Am J Med Genet 29:829–836

Reardon W, Smith A, Honour JW et al (2000) Evidence for digenic inheritance in some cases of Antley-Bixler syndrome? J Med Genet 37:26–32

Schinzel A, Savodelli G, Briner J, Sigg P, Massini C (1983) Antley-Bixler syndrome in sisters: a term newborn and a prenatally diagnosed fetus. Am J Med Genet 14:139–147

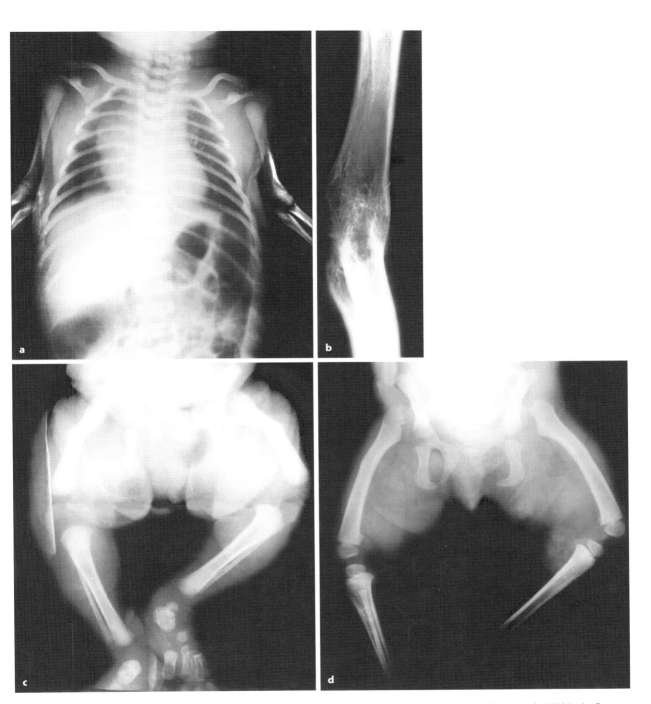

Fig. 3.22a–d. *Antley-Bixler syndrome.* **a** Newborn. Hypoplastic scapulae are seen. The elbow joints are not well visualized. **b** Same patient, 5 years. Distal humerus, proximal radius and ulna are completely fused. **c** Newborn The femora are bowed. There are no ossification centers in the knee epiphyses. **d** Four months. Within the first 4 months of life, the femora have spontaneously straightened. The ilia are long and narrow without acetabular fossae. The pubic and ischial bones are well ossified but narrow

Osteogenesis Imperfecta Types 2A and 3   MIM 166210, 259420

Synonym: Vrolik type of osteogenesis imperfecta.

Major Radiographic Features:
- Deficient calvarial ossification
- Generalized osteopenia
- Rib fractures, continuous in type 2 (thick ribs), discontinuous in type 3 (thin ribs)
- Deformed long bones, thick in type 2, thin and bowed with wide metaphyses in type 3
- Flattened vertebral bodies

Mode of Inheritance: Autosomal dominant; germinal or somatic mosaicism explaining multiple affected children of unaffected parents, resulting in an empiric recurrence risk of up to 7%.

Molecular Basis: Structural defects of type I collagen fibers resulting from mutations of the *COL1A1* gene on chromosome 17q21.31-q22.

Prenatal Diagnosis: Ultrasonography in the second trimester shows short, often bowed limbs, fractures, and increased nuchal translucency. Biochemical studies may show altered mobility of defective type I procollagen obtained from chorionic villi.

Differential Diagnosis: Severe cases with *osteogenesis imperfecta type 4* (caused by mutations of the *COL1A2* gene) may resemble type 3. The calvaria is usually better ossified in type 4, but biochemical or molecular studies may be necessary to differentiate the two conditions. The overall prognosis is better in type 4 than in type 3 osteogenesis imperfecta. *Osteogenesis 2C* is an extremely rare, autosomal recessive form of osteogenesis imperfecta manifesting with severely twisted, irregularly calcified long bones and ribs. Other types of osteogenesis imperfecta (types 1, 5, 6, 7) exist (Zeitlin et al. 2003) but are usually milder than types 2 and 3 at birth. Their differentiation requires biochemical and molecular studies. *Hypophosphatasia* differs by metaphyseal ossification defects, absence of wormian bones, and low alkaline phosphatase levels. Bone changes in the *Stüve-Wiedemann syndrome* and in *osteogenesis imperfecta type 1* are less severe. *Geroderma osteodysplasticum*, a rare disorder manifesting at birth with osteopenia, fractures, and wormian bones, is differentiated by the presence of wrinkled skin, sagging cheeks, and dislocated hips. Neonatal fractures occur in disorders with *thin diaphyses* including the various forms of *arthrogryposis*. Calvarial ossification is usually better preserved and the tubular bones are not as severely deformed as in osteogenesis imperfecta. Thin tubular bones and the presence of joint contractures allow one to differentiate these disorders. Neonatal joint contractures are also present in the *Bruck syndrome*, which otherwise resembles mild forms of osteogenesis imperfecta by the presence of neonatal fractures and wormian bones. The normal bone structure differentiates other forms of *congenital bowing* including *campomelic dysplasia, cartilage hair hypoplasia, dyssegmental dysplasias, Schwartz-Jampel syndrome,* and *Antley-Bixler syndrome*.

Prognosis: Most patients with the more severe type 2 (thick bone type) are stillborn or die within a few weeks after birth. Early mortality is also increased in type 3, but less severely affected patients may survive to adulthood. To some extent the individual prognosis can be predicted from a score based on the type and severity of bone changes (Spranger et al. 1982).

Remarks: Due to continuing fractures after birth, the appearance of the long bones can change within the first months of life from the thin, bowed diaphyses in type 3 to the thick tubular bones seen in newborns with type 2. Severe neonatal cases with osteogenesis imperfecta type 3 have also been classified as type 2B.

References

Chang LW, Chang CH, Yuu CH, Chang FM (2002) Three-dimensional ultrasonography of osteogenesis imperfecta at early pregnancy. Prenat Diagn 22:77–78

Cubert R, Cheng EY, Mack S, Pepin MG, Byers PH (2001) Osteogenesis imperfecta: mode of delivery and neonatal outcome. Obstet Gynecol 97:66–69

Leroy JG, Nuytinck L, de Paepe A et al (1998) Bruck syndrome: neonatal presentation and natural course in three patients. Pediatr Radiol 28:781–789

Ragunath M, Steinman B, Delozier-Blanchet C, Extermann P, Superti-Furga A (1994) Prenatal diagnosis of collagen disorders by direct biochemical analysis of chorionic villus biopsies. Pediatr Res 36:441–448

Shapiro JE, Phillips JA, Byers PH et al (1982) Prenatal diagnosis of lethal perinatal osteogenesis imperfecta (OI type II). J Pediatr 100:127–133

Sillence DO Barlow KK, Garber AP, Hall JC, Rimoin DL (1984) Osteogenesis imperfecta type II: delineation of the phenotype with reference to genetic heterogeneity. Am J Med Genet 17:407–423

Sillence DO, Barlow KK, Cole WG, Dietrich S, Garber AP, Rimoin DL (1986) Osteogenesis imperfecta type III: delineation of the phenotype with reference to genetic heterogeneity. Am J Med Genet 23:821–832

Spranger J, Cremin B, Beighton P (1982) Osteogenesis imperfecta congenita: features and prognosis of a heterogeneous condition. Pediatr Radiol 12:21–27

Zeitlin L, Fassier F, Glorieux FH (2003) Modern approach to children with osteogenesis imperfecta. J Pediatr Orthop 12:77–87

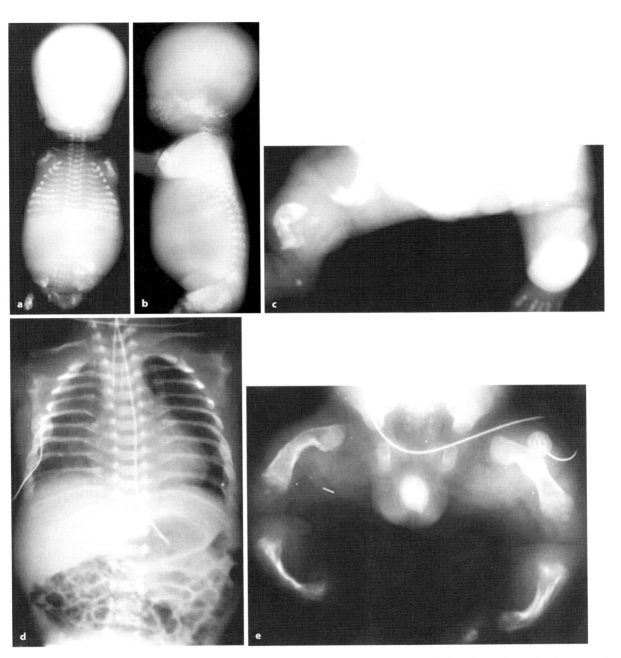

Fig. 3.23. *Osteogenesis imperfecta type 2.* **a–c** The calvarium is unossified. The ossified portions of the skeleton are undermineralized. The ribs are broad and irregular due to innumerable fractures. The vertebral bodies are flattened. The tubular bones are short, broad, crumpled, and bowed without diaphyseal constriction. **d, e** *Osteogenesis imperfecta type 3.* There is a generalized osteopenia. Multiple but discontinuous fractures are seen in the ribs. The tubular bones are short and bowed, but do not have the crumpled appearance of type 2

Infantile Hypophosphatasia   MIM 241500, 171760

Synonym: Rathbun disease

Major Radiographic Features:
- Absent ossification of major portions of the skull
- Poor ossification of the vertebrae; small scapulae and pelvic bones
- Short, thin ribs and tubular bones; absent ossification of whole bones
- Metaphyseal ossification defects reaching far into the diaphyses
- Occasionally bone spurs extending from the midshafts of long tubular bones (Bowdler spurs)

Mode of Inheritance: Autosomal recessive.

Molecular Basis: Mutations of the *TNSALP* gene located on chromosome 1p36.1-p34 encoding the tissue-nonspecific alkaline phosphatase; compound heterozygosity or homozygosity of mutated *TNSALP* genes resulting in infantile hypophosphatasia; mutations of the *TNSALP* gene sometimes expressing in the heterozygous state, leading to the milder manifestations of childhood or adult hypophosphatasia, with autosomal dominant inheritance.

Prenatal Diagnosis: Ultrasonography may reveal absent ossification of the calvaria, bowed legs, and increased nuchal translucency at 12–14 weeks' gestation. An affected fetus may be identified by determination of alkaline phosphatase activity in chorionic villi, in culture amniotic cells, or in fetal blood obtained by cordocentesis. If the TNSALP mutation is known from a previous affected child, mutational analysis in fetal cells is possible.

Differential Diagnosis: *Osteogenesis imperfecta* differs by the presence of rib fractures and absence of metaphyseal lesions. Various forms of *achondrogenesis* are differentiated by the tubular bones being short and thick, rather than thin. The metaphyseal lesions in the *Sedaghatian type of lethal chondrodysplasias* are not associated with the severe demineralization characterizing hypophos-phatasia. Bowing of the long bones, Bowdler spurs, and low alkaline phosphatase have been observed in *cleidocranial dysplasia*. However, the clavicles are hypoplastic, and undermineralization is less severe in that disorder than in infantile hypophosphatasia.

Prognosis: Severe infantile hypophosphatasia is lethal, mostly due to respiratory compromise, failure to thrive, and other signs of hypercalcemia (sometimes convulsions occur).

Remarks: Diagnostic aids in newborns with suggested hypophosphatasia are the low activity of serum alkaline phosphatase, elevated urinary excretion of phosphoethanolamine, and elevated plasma concentration of pyridoxal 5' phosphate. Serum alkaline phosphatase activity may be low in the parents.

References

Litmanovitz RO, Dolfin T, Arnon S et al (2002) Glu2478Lys/ Gly309Arg mutation of the tissue-nonspecific alkaline phosphatase gene in neonatal hypophosphatasia associated with convulsions. J Inherit Metab Dis 25:35–40

Mornet E, Taillandier A, Peyramaure S et al (1998) Identification of fifteen novel mutations in the tissue-nonspecific alkaline phosphatase (TNSALP) gene in European patients with severe hypophosphatasia. Eur J Hum Genet 6:308–314

Pauli RM, Modaff P, Sipes S, Whyte MP (1999) Mild hypophosphatasia mimicking severe osteogenesis imperfecta in utero: bent but not broken. Am J Med Genet 86:434–438

Sergi C, Mornet E, Troeger J, Voigtlaender T (2001) Perinatal hypophosphatasia: radiology, pathology and molecular biology studies in a family harboring a splicing mutation (648+1A) and a novel missense mutation (N400S) in the tissue-nonspecific alkaline phosphatase (TNSALP) gene. Am J Med Genet 103:235–240

Souka AP Raymond FL, Mornet E, Geerts L, Nicolaides KH (2002) Hypophosphatasia associated with increased nuchal translucency: a report of two affected pregnancies. Ultrasound Obstet Gynecol 20:294–295

Stoll C, Fischbach M, Terzic J et al (2002) Severe hyphosphatasia due to mutations in the tissue-nonspecific alkaline phosphatase (TNSALP) gene. Genet Couns 13:289–29

Unger S, Mornet E, Mundlos S, Blaser S, Cole DE (2002) Severe cleidocranial dysplasia can mimic hypophosphatasia. Eur J Pediatr 161:623–626

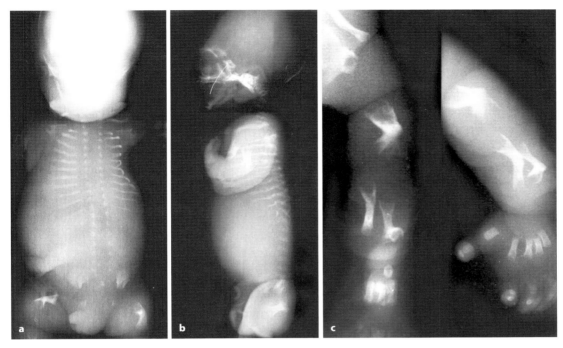

Fig. 3.24a–c. *Infantile Hypophosphatasia severe form.* Stillborn, 27 weeks' gestation. **a, b** Calvaria, mandibulae and vertebral bodies are not ossified. The ribs are short, thin, and irregularly ossified. **c** The tubular bones are short and bowed with V-shaped ossification defects at their ends reaching deep into the diaphyses

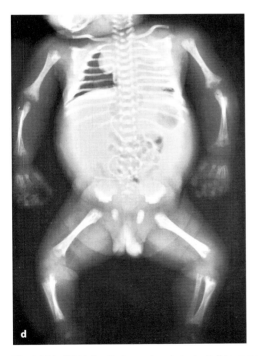

Fig. 3.24d. *Mild infantile hypophosphatasia.* Full-term neonate. The ribs are thin. The lower lumbar and sacral vertebral bodies are small and the pubic bones are not ossified. The tubular bones are straight and well modeled with punched-out metaphyseal ossification defects

Jansen Metaphyseal Dysplasia   MIM 156400

Synonym: Metaphyseal chondrodysplasia, Murk Jansen type.

Major Radiographic Features:
- Generalized demineralization, occasionally fractures
- Splayed ribs ends
- Metaphyseal cupping and fraying of tubular bones

Mode of Inheritance: Autosomal dominant.

Molecular Basis: Mutations of the *PTHR1* gene located on chromosome 3p22-p22.1 result in a constitutive activation of the receptor for the parathyroid hormone/parathyroid-hormone-related protein (PTHR1) in pre-hypertrophic chondrocytes of the growth plate. This interferes with the differentiation of chondrocytes and subsequent bone formation.

Prenatal Diagnosis: Affected children may be normal at birth and not be recognized by fetal ultrasound. Short limbs and defective calvarial ossification may be seen in others. In familial cases, molecular analysis may be attempted.

Differential Diagnosis: In *hypophosphatasia* the metaphyseal defects are more regular and the undermineralization is usually more severe. *Infantile rickets* are excluded by low calcium and elevated alkaline phosphatase. Cortical erosion, increased subperiosteal bone formation, and metaphyseal irregularities occur in isolated *neonatal hyperparathyroidism* and in hyperparathyroidism associated with *mucolipidosis II*. Biochemical tests may be needed to rule out these conditions. In *Sedaghatian metaphyseal dysplasia* bone mineralization is not defective.

Prognosis: Life expectancy and mental development are normal.

Remarks: Absence of a functional receptor for PTH/PTHR1 receptor results in Blomstrand dysplasia.

References

Charrow J, Poznanski AK (1984) The Jansen type of metaphyseal chondrodysplasia: confirmation of dominant inheritance and review of radiographic manifestations in the newborn and adult. Am J Med Genet 18:321–327

Schipani E, Kruse K, Jüppner H (1995) A constitutively active mutant PTH-PTHrH receptor in Jansen type metaphyseal chondrodysplasia. Science 268:989–100

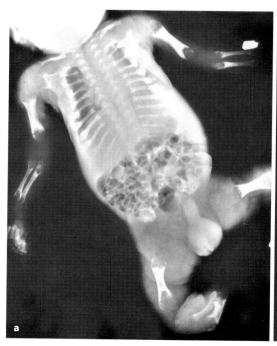
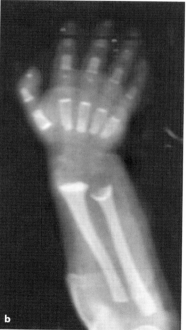

Fig. 3.25a, b. *Jansen type of metaphyseal dysplasia*, 36 weeks' gestation. **a, b** The tubular bones and ribs are short with large, relatively uniform, hollowed-out metaphyseal lesions. Pubic and ischial bones are not ossified. Ossification of the vertebral bodies is defective. Cortical bone erosion and excessive subperiosteal bone formation are not present in this patient

Stüve-Wiedemann Syndrome   MIM 601559

Synonym: Schwartz-Jampel syndrome, type 2.

Major Radiographic Features:
- Bowing of the long tubular bones with internal cortical thickening
- Generalized rarefaction
- Enlarged, radiolucent metaphyses

Mode of Inheritance: Autosomal recessive.

Prenatal Diagnosis: (Nonspecific) bowing of the long bones has been detected by ultrasound in the 22nd week of gestation.

Differential Diagnosis: Bowing of the long bones is nonspecific. Bowing disorders without osteopenia are differentiated by the normal bone structure (see *campomelic dysplasia*). The various forms of *osteogenesis imperfecta* are associated with defective calvarial ossification, rib fractures, and fractures of the tubular bones. Severely deficient ossification and punched-out metaphyseal lesions characterize *hypophosphatasia*.

Prognosis: Most patients die in infancy, failing to thrive and exhibiting recurrent episodes of unexplained fever. Patients have been described who survived into mid-childhood with progressing bowing, spinal deformities, and neurological symptoms including temperature instability, reduced pain sensation, and absent corneal and patellar reflexes. Mentality was normal.

Remarks: In spite of some clinical and osseous similarities, the Schwartz-Jampel syndrome and Stüve-Wiedemann syndrome are distinct genetic disorders.

References

Al-Gazali LI, Ravenscroit A, Feng A et al (2003) Stuve-Wiedemann syndrome in children surviving infancy: clinical and radiological features. Clin Dysmorphol 12:1–8

Cormier-Daire V, Superti-Furga A, Munnich A et al (1998) Clinical homogeneity of the Stüve-Wiedemann syndrome and overlap with the Schwartz-Jampel syndrome type 2. Am J Med Genet 78:146–149

Farra C, Piquet C, Guillaume M, D'Ercole C, Philip N (2002) Congenital bowing of long bones: prenatal ultrasound findings and diagnostic dilemmas. Fetal Diagn Ther 17:236–239

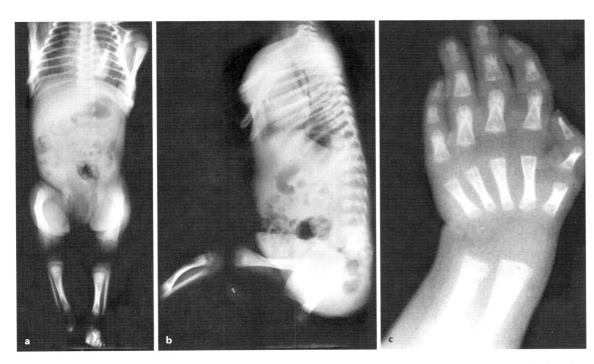

Fig. 3.26a–c. *Stüve-Wiedemann syndrome*. a The ribs are thin. The femora are bowed with wide, radiolucent metaphyses and increased cortical thickness of the diaphyses. Dense diaphyses and widened, radiolucent metaphyses create a bishop's-miter-like configuration of the bone ends. **b** The vertebral bodies are rounded but their height is not decreased. Metaphyseal widening is seen in the distal femur and the tibia. **c** Note miter-like configuration of the tubular bones, best seen in the proximal phalanges. (Illustrations courtesy of Dr. P. Meinecke, Hamburg)

Oto-palato-digital Syndrome Type II   MIM 304120

Synonym: OPD-II; Cranio-oro-digital syndrome.

Major Radiographic Features:
- Poorly ossified calvaria with dense skull base and prominent supraorbital ridges
- Thin, sinuous ribs
- Bowed long tubular bones; sometimes fibula a/hypoplasia
- Short, squared, irregularly formed short tubular bones; often a/hypoplasia of the first and second digits

Mode of Inheritance: X-linked dominant, with severe expression in males, mostly mild or minimal in females.

Molecular Basis: Mutations of *FLNA* located on Xq28 encoding filamin A, a protein regulating the actin cytoskeleton.

Prenatal Diagnosis: Bowed tubular bones, small chest and/or boy wall defects are found by sonography.

Differential Diagnosis: OPD-II shows considerable overlap with *OPD-I* and *Melnick-Needles syndrome* but differs by the more severe bone changes and early lethality (see "Remarks"). Multiple dislocations are more common in the *Larsen syndrome* than in OPD-II. OPD is X-linked, the Larsen syndrome autosomal dominant. In the *Yunis-Varon syndrome* the tubular bones are thin but not bowed and the clavicles are hypoplastic or absent. Broad, squared metacarpals and phalanges are seen in mild expressions of *atelosteogenesis,* which differ by the distal hypoplasia of the femora and humeri and the absence of bowing deformities. *Campomelic dysplasia* and *other bowing syndromes without osteopenia* are differentiated by their milder manifestations, notably their more normal ribs and short tubular bones

Prognosis: The prognosis varies depending on the severity of the clinical manifestations. Lethality is increased due to respiratory insufficiency and associated rare malformations including tracheal stenosis and hydrocephaly, and cardiac, ventral wall, or neural tube defects.

Remarks: OPD-II is at the severe end of a clinical spectrum including OPD-I, the Melnick-Needles syndrome, and frontometaphyseal dysplasia, all of which are caused by allelic mutations of the *FNLA* gene leading to varying degrees of up-regulation of filamin and ensuing abnormalities of the cytoskeleton. Note the pathogenetic and phenotypic relationships between the OPD family of disorders caused by filamin A defects and the Atelosteogenesis/Larsen family of disorders caused by defects of filamin B. Both filamins are involved in the organization of the cytoskeleton.

References

Robertson SP, Gunn T, Allen B, Chapman C, Becroft D (1997) Are Melnick-Needles syndrome and otopalato-digital syndrome type II allelic? Am J Med Genet 71:341–347

Robertson SP, Twigg SRF, Sutherland-Smith AJ et al (2003) Localized mutations in FLNA, encoding the actin cross-linking protein filamin A cause diverse malformations in humans (in press)

Savarirayan R, Cormier-Daire V, Unger S et al (2000) Oto-palato-digital syndrome, type II: report of three cases with further delineation of the chondro-osseous morphology. Am J Med Genet 95:193–200

Verloes A, Lesenfants S, Barr M et al (2000) Fronto-oto-palato-digital osteodysplasia: Clinical evidence for a single entity encompassing Melnick-Needles syndrome, otopalatodigital syndrome types 1 and 2, and frontometaphyseal dysplasia. Am J Med Genet 90:407–422

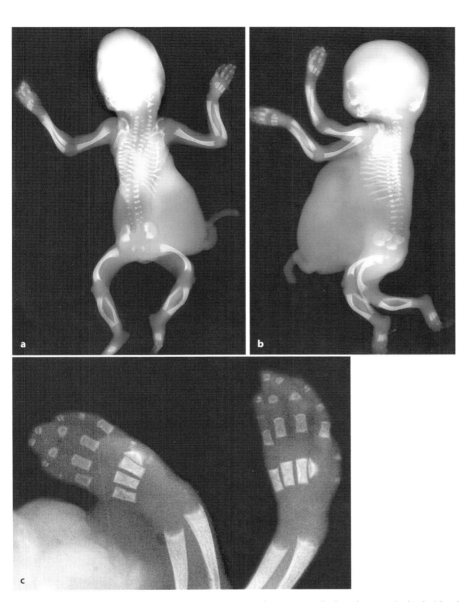

Fig. 3.27a–c. *Oto-palato-digital syndrome type II*, 18 weeks' gestation. **a** The chest is small with 11 thin, ribbon-like ribs. The long tubular bones are bowed. **b** The skull film shows a well ossified base with a prominent frontal torus and absent ossification of the calvaria. The vertebral bodies are small. Coronal clefts are present in the upper lumbar bodies. Note sinuous appearance of the ribs and bowing of the long bones. **c** On both sides the thumbs are hypoplastic with tiny ossification centers in the metacarpal and proximal phalanx. Bilaterally, the second metacarpals are small and crescent shaped. The metacarpals and proximal phalanges of the 2nd to 5th digits are short and squared, the middle and distal phalanges very short and distally pointed

Fetal Apokinesia/Hypokinesia Sequence   MI 208150, 300073

Synonyms: Includes Pena-Shokeir syndrome, arthrogryposes.

Major Radiographic Features:
- Thin ribs
- Thin tubular bones without metaphyseal enlargement
- Often fractures

Etiopathogenesis: Intrauterine mobility of the fetus may be impeded by numerous genetic and nongenetic factors. Causes limiting fetal mobility fall into six categories (modified from Hall 2002):
1. Neuropathic processes, central or peripheral
2. Myopathic processes including congenital myopathies
3. Intrauterine exposure to immobilizing substances including curare, haloperidol
4. Maternal illness including infections and compromise of blood supply to the fetus
5. Connective tissue or skin diseases restricting joint mobility
6. External limitation of space including oligohydramnios, twinning, abnormal uterus

Restriction of fetal movement for extended periods results in a nonspecific clinical phenotype encompassing multiple joint contractures, pterygia, micrognathia, pulmonary hypoplasia, short umbilical cord, and growth retardation. If the hypomobility is caused by decreased fetal muscle activity (categories 1–4), bone modeling and periosteal bone apposition are decreased, and thin ribs and tubular bones become part of the fetal a/hypokinesia sequence. If the intrauterine muscle stress remains normal (categories 5, 6), such as in the Potter sequence and other disorders associated with oligohydramnios, the ribs and tubular bones develop normally.

Prenatal Diagnosis: Decreased intrauterine mobility may be detected in the 2nd trimester by real-time ultrasound. Depending on the specific condition, associated malformations may be detected.

Differential Diagnosis: The fetal akinesia sequence is a secondary deformation syndrome asking for a primary diagnosis. *"Osteocraniostenosis"* differs by the abrupt metaphyseal flare of the thin tubular bones. In *microcephalic osteodysplastic primordial dwarfism* the tubular bones are slender but not as thin as in fetal akinesia and not associated with fractures.

Prognosis: It depends on the primary cause. Thin tubular bones and ribs point to long-standing intrauterine hypomobility implying a guarded prognosis.

Remarks: The term "arthrogryposis" refers nonspecifically to multiple joint contractures associated with intrauterine a/hypokinesia. The distinction of different forms of arthrogryposis and their association with specific morphological abnormalities help elucidate the underlying cause. Associated with the sequelae of intrauterine hypomobility may be morphologic manifestations of the primary disorder such as cerebral, eye, cardiac, or renal defects.

The "Pena-Shokair syndrome, type I" is the hypokinesia sequence caused by a hereditary motor neuropathy. The term "Pena-Shokair syndrome type II" refers to a cerebro-ocular disorder leading to intrauterine hypokinesia and its ensuing deformation sequence.

References
Chen H, Blackburn WR, Wertelecki W (1995) Fetal akinesia and multiple perinatal fractures. Am J Med Genet 55:273–477

Hall JG (2001) Arthrogryposes (multiple congenital contractures). In: Rimoin DL, Connor JM, Pyeritz RE, Korf BR (eds) Principles and practice of medical genetics, 4th edn. Churchill Livingstone, London, pp 4182–42

Palacios J, Rodriguez JI (1990) Extrinsic fetal akinesia and skeletal development: a study in oligohydramnios sequence. Teratology 42:1–5

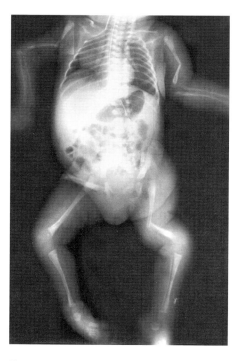

Fig. 3.28. *Fetal a/hypokinesia sequence.* Newborn, 36 weeks' gestation, with lissencephaly, severe intrauterine hypotonia, multiple joint contractures, micrognathia, pulmonary hypoplasia. Ribs and clavicles are thin; the vertebral bodies are well developed. The long tubular bones are thin, poorly modeled but not bowed. Multiple fractures

Osteocraniostenosis   MIM 602361

Major Radiographic Features:

- Cloverleaf, acrocephalic or brachycephalic skull configuration; deficient calvarial ossification
- Very thin tubular bones with abrupt metaphyseal flare
- Hypoplasia of the distal phalanges

Mode of Inheritance: Unknown, possibly dominant.

Molecular Basis: Unknown.

Prenatal Diagnosis: Thin tubular bones with or without fractures and cranial abnormalities are prenatally detected by ultrasound.

Differential Diagnosis: Patients with the *a/hypokinesia sequence* lack the abrupt metaphyseal flare of the tubular bones and usually have associated joint contractures and other manifestations of intrauterine hypomobility. Chondro-osseous histology is normal in fetal a/hypokinesia and abnormal in osteocraniostenosis. In *gracile bone dysplasia* bone density is decreased, metaphyseal widening of the tubular bones is absent or minimal. and there are no cranial deformities.

Prognosis: Affected infants were stillborn or died shortly after birth.

Remarks: Gracile bone dysplasia and osteocraniostenosis have been lumped as one entity (MIM 602361). However, the two conditions differ sufficiently to consider them as separate entities. Osteocraniostenosis is characterized by an abnormal cranium, a/hyposplenia, abrupt metaphyseal flare, and abnormalities of the endochondral bone formation. Gracile bone dysplasia is characterized by a small but otherwise normal cranium, intracerebral calcifications, stick-like tubular bones with little or no metaphyseal flare, ischial hypoplasia, and overgrowth of cortical bone. In both conditions the osseous abnormalities appear to be primary manifestations of pleiotropic mutations, i.e., dysplasias, whereas in the fetal a/hypokinesia sequence they are secondary deformations.

References

Costa T, Azouz EM, Fitzpatrick J et al (1998) Skeletal dysplasia with gracile bones: Three new cases, including two offspring of a mother with a dwarfing condition. Am J Med Genet 76:125–132 (family B)

Kozlowski K, Masel J, Sillence DO, Arbuckle S, Juttnerova V (2002) Gracile bone dysplasias. Pediatr Radiol 32:629– 634 (cases 1 and 2)

Maroteaux P, Cohen-Solal L, Bonaventure J et al (1988) Syndromes létaux avec gracilité du squelette. Arch Franç Pediatr 45: 477–481 (cases 5 and 6)

Verloes A, Narcy F, Grattagliano B et al (1994) Osteocraniostenosis. J Med Genet 31:772–778

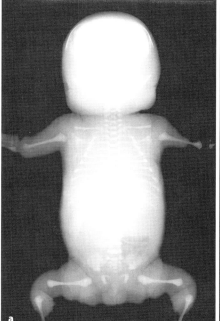
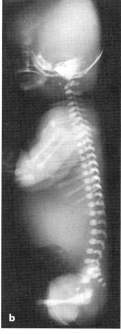

Fig. 3.29a, b. *Osteocraniostenosis,* 38 weeks' gestation. There is a cloverleaf deformity of the skull. The ribs are thin and slightly irregular. The shafts of the long tubular bones are thin with a characteristically abrupt metaphyseal flare. Note normally developed vertebral bodies and normal bone density. (Courtesy of Dr. K. Runge, Wuppertal)

Gracile Bone Dysplasia   MIM 602361

Major Radiographic Features:

- Thin ribs and clavicles
- Deficient ossification of pubic and ischial bones
- Short and slender, stick-like tubular bones with lack of cortical demarcation

Mode of Inheritance: Probably autosomal recessive.

Molecular Basis: Unknown.

Prenatal Diagnosis: Short limbs are detected by sonography.

Differential Diagnosis: Joint contractures and other manifestations of intrauterine hypomobility are conspicuous in *fetal a/hypokinesia*. In that condition tubular bone modeling is better preserved and chondro-osseous histology is normal. The stick-like appearance of the tubular bones and absence of gross cranial deformities differentiate gracile bone dysplasia from *osteocraniostenosis*.

Prognosis: All infants were stillborn or died shortly after birth due to respiratory insufficiency.

Remarks: Although osteocraniostenosis and gracile bone dysplasia have been lumped as one condition (MIM 602361), radiographic and histologic differences exist that allow their provisional separation as discrete entities (see "Osteocraniostenosis"). The term "gracile bone dysplasias" has also been used as a generic term to denote all neonatal disorders with slender bones (Kozlowski et al. 2002).

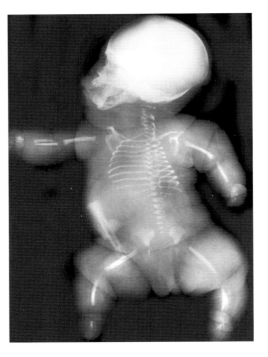

Fig. 3.30. *Gracile bone dysplasia,* full-term newborn. The chest is small and the ribs are thin. Note the well-ossified calvaria and clavicles. The lower portions of the ilia and the ischial bones are hypoplastic and the pubic bones are not ossified. The tubular bones are shortened and gracile but with relatively wide mid portions and lack of metaphyseal flare

References

Kozlowski K, Masel J, Sillence DO, Arbuckle S, Juttnerova V (2002) Gracile bone dysplasias. Pediatr Radiol 32:629–634 (cases 1 and 2)

Thomas JA, Rimoin DL, Lachman RS, Wilcox WR (1998) Gracile bone dysplasia. Am J Med Genet 75:95–100

Microcephalic Osteodysplastic Primordial Dwarfism, Type I   MIM 210710, 210720, 210730

Synonym: MOD-1 Osteodysplastic primordial dwarfism, Taybi-Linder syndrome, cephaloskeletal dysplasia, brachymelic primordial dwarfism; includes microcephalic osteodysplastic primordial dwarfism, type 3.

Major Radiographic Features:
- Microcephaly with sloping forehead
- Short, broad ilia
- Shortened, slender tubular bones with preserved modeling

Mode of Inheritance: Autosomal recessive.

Prenatal Diagnosis: Short limbs may be detected by ultrasound.

Differential Diagnosis: In the fetal *hypokinesia sequence, osteocraniostenosis,* and *gracile bone dysplasia* the tubular bones are thinner (more fishbone-like) than in MOD-1. In contrast to *other forms of primordial dwarfism*, dwarfism is disproportionate in MOD-1. The *Kenny-Caffey syndrome* is differentiated by the increased cortical thickness, medullary stenosis, and hypocalcemia. It is rarely manifested at birth.

Prognosis: Early mortality is increased. Surviving infants suffer from recurrent apneas, seizures, and psychomotor retardation. The patients fail to develop both physically and mentally. Death usually occurs before one year of age, mostly from intercurrent infections.

Remarks: The bone changes in MOD-1 are nonspecific and occur also in other forms of primordial dwarfism, including MOD-2, Silver-Russel-syndrome, 3 M syndrome, and others. The prognosis is much better in most of these latter disorders and the connatal dwarfism is proportionate. The absence of microcephaly with a receding forehead cautions against a diagnosis of MOD-1.

References
Majewski F, Spranger J (1976) Über einen neuen Typ des primordialen Minderwuchses: der brachymele primordiale Minderwuchs. Monatsschr Kinderheilkd 124:499–503

Meinecke, Schaefer E, Wiedemann HR (1991) Microcephalic osteodysplastic primordial dwarfism: further evidence for identity of the so-called types I and III. Am J Med Genet 39:232–236

Sigaudy S, Toutain A, Moncla A et al (1998) Microcephalic osteodysplastic primordial dwarfism Taybi-Linder type: report of four cases and review of the literature. Am J Med Genet 80:16–24

Spranger JW, Brill PWE, Poznanski A (2002) Bone dysplasia, 2nd edn., Elsevier GmbH, Urban & Fischer, Munich

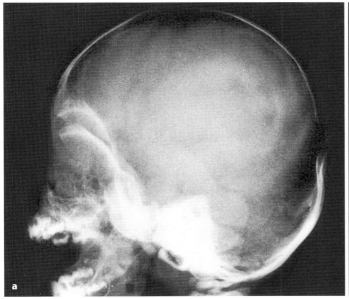
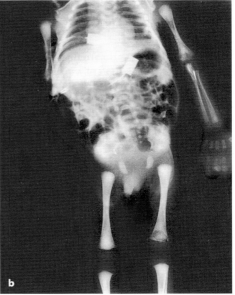

Fig. 3.31a, b. *Microcephalic osteodysplastic primordial dwarfism, type 1.* **a** The skull is small and brachycephalic with a receding forehead, steep base, and almost closed anterior fontanelle. **b** The ilia are short due to hypoplasia of the lower portions. The pubic bones are not ossified. The long bones are short and slender but well modeled. (From: Spranger et al.: Bone Dysplasias, 2nd edn., 2002, with kind permission from Elsevier GmbH, Urban & Fischer, Munich)

Mucolipidosis II   MIM 252500

Synonym: I-cell-disease; Leroy disease.

Major Radiographic Features:
- Decreased bone mineralization
- Foreshortened vertebral bodies, sometimes butterfly vertebrae
- Metaphyseal cupping and fraying of the tubular bones
- Excessive periosteal new bone formation and diaphyseal expansion of the long tubular bones
- Pelvic dysplasia
- Occasionally punctate calcifications and bone defects

Mode of Inheritance: Autosomal recessive.

Molecular Basis: Mutations of a gene on chromosome 4q21–23 encoding phosphotransferase.

Prenatal Diagnosis: Once the diagnosis is suspected on the basis of an older affected sibling, the disorder can be diagnosed in the 2nd trimester by demonstrating decreased activity of multiple lysosomal enzymes in chorionic cells or cultured amniotic cells. Lysosomal enzymes are increased in amniotic fluid. Fetal hydrops is often present.

Differential Diagnosis: The skeletal abnormalities in *GM₁ gangliosidosis* are very similar to those in mucoli-

pidosis II, and the two disorders are differentiated by biochemical analysis showing isolated deficiency of β-galactosidase in the former and deficient activity of multiple lysosomal enzymes in the latter. Fetal hydrops is a nonspecific manifestation of multiple *lysosomal storage diseases* including mucopolysaccharidoses types I, VII, infantile sialidosis, galactosialidosis, and infantile free sialic acid storage disease. In these disorders the neonatal bone changes are those of comparatively mild dysostosis multiplex, without periosteal cloaking and metaphyseal fraying and cupping. The tubular bone abnormalities often suggest a diagnosis of *neonatal rickets* or neonatal *hyperparathyroidism*. Wide ribs and pelvic dysplasia are not seen in these disorders and lysosomal enzyme activities are normal.

References

Carey WF, Jaunzems A, Richardson M, Fong BA, Chin SJ, Nelson PV (1999) Prenatal diagnosis of mucolipidosis II – electron microscopy and biochemical evaluation. Prenat Diagn 19:525–526

Herman TE, McAlister WH (1996) Neonatal mucolipidosis II (I-cell disease) with dysharmonic epiphyseal ossification and butterfly vertebral body. J Perinatol 16:400–402

Pazzaglia UE, Beluffi G, Danesino C et al (1989) Neonatal mucolipidosis 2. The spontaneous evolution of early bone lesions and the effect of vitamin D treatment. Pediatr Radiol 20:80–84

Stone DL, Sidransky E (1999) Hydrops fetalis: lysosomal storage disorders in extremis. Adv Pediatr 46:409–440

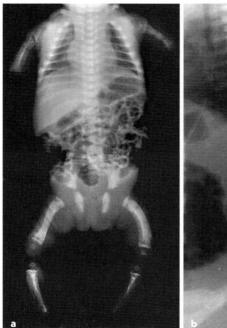
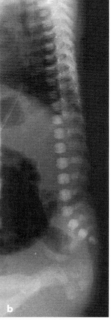

Fig. 3.32a, b. *Mucolipidosis II,* full-term newborn. **a** The femora are thick and bowed with a coarsely woven bone structure and periosteal cloaking. These changes are reminiscent of those in neonatal hyperparathyroidism. The lower ilia are hypoplastic with a wide iliac angle. **b** The vertebral bodies are foreshortened

Pacman Dysplasia   MIM 167220

Major Radiographic Features:
- Shortened tubular bones
- Abnormal bone structure with irregular, coarsely woven trabeculation, deficient cortical bone formation, and metaphyseal hyperdensities; periosteal cloaking in some patients
- Deficient cortical bone formation
- Flattened vertebral bodies with coronal clefts
- Femoral bowing
- Punctate calcifications

Mode of Inheritance: Probably autosomal recessive.

Prenatal Diagnosis: Short, deformed tubular bones detectable by sonography at 16 weeks' gestation.

Differential Diagnosis: Neonatal *hyperparathyroidism* manifests with coarse bone trabeculation, but not with punctuate calcifications and platyspondyly. Calcific stippling is more extensive in the various forms of *chondrodysplasia punctata*. Punctate calcifications are nonspecific findings in numerous disorders that, in contrast to Pacman dysplasia, do not show the coarsely woven, irregular bone structure seen in this condition.

Prognosis: All known patients were aborted because of prenatally detected skeletal abnormalities.

Remarks: A sibling born to a patient with Pacman dysplasia survived the neonatal period and was biochemically and clinically proven to have mucolipidosis II (Saul R, personal communication 2004). Thus Pacman dysplasia is a variant manifestation of Mucolipidosis II.

References

Miller SF, Proud VK, Werner AL et al (2003) Pacman dysplasia: a lethal skeletal dysplasia with variable radiographic features. Pediatr Radiol 33:256–260

Shoat M, Rimoin DL, Gruber HE, Lachman R (1993) New epiphyseal stippling syndrome with osteoclastic hyperplasia. Am J Med Genet 45:558–561

Wilcox WR, Lucas BC, Loebel B et al (1998) Pacman dysplasia: report of two affected sibs. Am J Med Genet 77:272–276

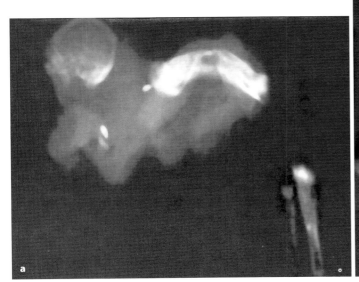
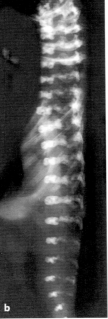

Fig. 3.33a, b. *Pacman dysplasia,* 21 weeks gestation. **a** The femur is short and bowed with coarse, irregular trabeculation, deficient cortical bone, and metaphyseal hyperdensity. The ileum is round and undermineralized except for the supraacetabular region. Tibiae and fibula are osteopenic except for the dense tibial metaphysis. **b** The vertebral bodies are flat with an irregular bone structure and coronal clefts in the thoracic region. (Reproduced from Wilcox et al. 1998, by permission of first author and publisher)

Infantile Cortical Hyperostosis   MIM 114000

Synonyms: Caffey-Silverman disease; Caffey disease; Roske-Caffey disease.

Major Radiographic Features:
- Cortical hyperostosis of single or multiple bones
- In severe cases, short and bowed tubular bones

Mode of Inheritance: Autosomal dominant. One parent may have had the disorder in infancy with complete resolution making proper genetic counseling difficult.

Prenatal Diagnosis: In severe cases, short, bowed limbs with thickened, irregularly echodense diaphyses may be detected by ultrasound. Fetal hydrops and polyhydramnios may be present.

Differential Diagnosis: Other *bowing disorders* including osteogenesis imperfecta and hypophosphatasia do not show the dense, irregularly widened diaphyses. *Mucolipidosis II* is differentiated by the generalized osteopenia, pelvic dysplasia, and abnormal vertebral bodies. *Secondary hyperostoses* occur in conjunction with infections, in scurvy and rickets, after prostaglandin E administration, and in cardiopulmonary disorders, but are not present perinatally.

Prognosis: Severely affected cases may be stillborn or die at birth of respiratory failure. The prognosis is good in mildly affected patients with isolated lesions, mostly in clavicles, mandible, ulnae, ribs, or scapulae. In most of these cases complete clinical and radiographic recovery can be expected within weeks or months.

References

De Jong G, Muller LMM (1995) Perinatal death in two sibs with infantile cortical hyperostosis (Caffey disease). Am J Med Genet 59: 134–138

Lecolier B, Bercau G, Gonzales M et al (1992) Radiographic, haematological, and biochemical findings in a fetus with Caffey disease. Prenatal Diag 12:637–641

MacLachlan AK, Gerrard JW, Houston CS, Ives EJ (1984) Familial infantile cortical hyperostosis in a large Canadian family. Canad Med Assoc J 130:1172–1174

Stevenson RE (1993) Findings of heritable Caffey disease on ultrasound at 35 1/2 weeks' gestation. Proc Green Genet Ctr 12: 16–18

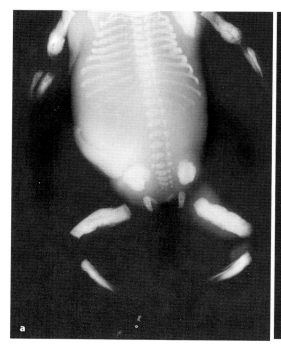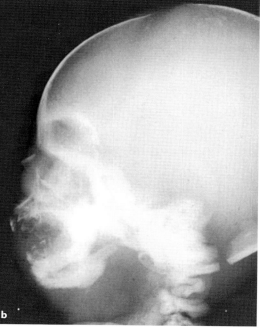

Fig. 3.34a, b. *Infantile cortical hyperostosis;* 23 weeks' gestation. **a** The long tubular bones are shortened and thickened due to excessive masses of cortical bone. There is mild anterior bossing of the tibiae. **b** Cortical hyperostosis is seen in the mandible

Short Rib (-Polydactyly) Syndrome, Saldino-Noonan/Verma-Naumoff Type

MIM 263530,
MIM 263510

Synonym: Includes short rib (-polydactyly) type I (Saldino-Noonan) and Short rib-polydactyly syndrome III (Verma Naumoff); SRPS-I and SRPS-III.

Major Radiographic Features:

- Short, horizontally oriented ribs
- Small iliac bones with horizontal acetabular roofs
- Shortness of tubular bones with a pointed (torpedo-like) or ragged (banana-peel-like) appearance
- Postaxial polydactyly in most cases

Mode of Inheritance: Autosomal recessive.

Prenatal Diagnosis: Sonography shows short tubular bones and short ribs, sometimes pancreatic cysts.

Differential Diagnosis: In the *Beemer-Langer* and *Majewski types* of short rib (-polydactyly) syndrome the pelvis has a more normal appearance and the ends of the tubular bones are smooth. In *asphyxiating thoracic dysplasia* the long bones are less severely affected. Patients with *Chondroectodermal dysp*lasia (Ellis-van Creveld syndrome) have a more normal thorax and progressive proximal-distal shortening of the extremities.

Prognosis: The patients are stillborn or die shortly after birth from cardiorespiratory insufficiency.

Remarks: The long bone changes in the Saldino-Noonan type are slightly more severe than in the Verma-Naumoff-Type. However, torpedo-like and banana-peel-like lesions can occur in the same patient and are probably the expression of allelic mutations.

References

Martinez-Frias ML, Bermejo E, Urioste M, Huertas H, Arrozo I (1993) Lethal short rib-polydactyly syndromes: further evidence for their overlapping in a continuous spectrum . J Med Genet 30: 937

Sarafoglou K, Funai EF, Fefferman N et al (1999) Short rib-polydactyly syndrome: more evidence of a continuous spectrum. Clin Genet 56:145–148

Spranger JW, Brill PWE, Poznanski A (2002) Bone dysplasias, 2nd edn. Urban-Fischer, Oxford

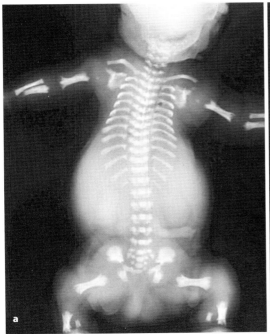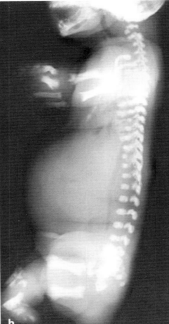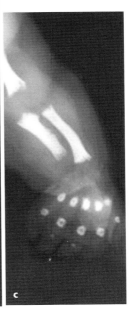

Fig. 3.35a–c. *Short rib (-polydactyly), Saldino-Noonan/Verma-Naumoff type,* 35 weeks' gestation. **a** There is a striking restriction of the thoracic cage caused by very short and horizontally oriented ribs. The scapulae are small with irregular margins. The ilia are small with horizontal inferior margins, and small triangular ossification defects are seen above their lateral aspects. The tubular bones are short with spurs of none extending longitudinally from the medial and lateral aspects of the metaphyses resulting in a banana-peel appearance. **b** The vertebral bodies are small with irregular upper and lower margins and absent ossification in the cervical spine. **c** Metacarpals and proximal phalanges are very small; the middle and distal phalanges are not ossified except for two tiny ossification centers in the middle phalanges of digits 3 and 4. Note short radius and ulna with longitudinal spurs extending from the lateral and medial aspects of the bone ends

Short Rib (-Polydactyly) Syndrome, Beemer-Langer Type   MIM 269860

Synonym: Short rib syndrome, Beemer-Langer type; Beemer-Langer syndrome; Short rib (-polydactyly) syndrome, type IV; SRPS IV.

Major Radiographic Features:
- Short, horizontally oriented ribs
- Small iliac bones
- Shortened tubular bones with smooth ends
- Tibia not essentially shorter than fibula
- Bowed radius and ulna
- Polydactyly in some patients

Mode of Inheritance: Autosomal recessive.

Prenatal Diagnosis: Sonography shows short tubular bones and short ribs.

Differential Diagnosis: The metaphyseal margins are irregular in the *Saldino-Noonan/Verma-Naumoff type*. In the *Majewski type* of short rib (-polydactyly) syndrome the tibiae is shorter than the fibula. In *asphyxiating thoracic dysplasia* the long bones are less severely affected. Patients with *Chondroectodermal dysp*lasia (Ellis-van Creveld syndrome) have a more normal thorax and progressive proximal-distal shortening of the extremities.

Prognosis: The patients are stillborn or die shortly after birth from cardiorespiratory insufficiency.

References
Elcioglu N, Karatekin G, Sezgin B, Nuhoglu A, Cenani A (1996) Short rib-polydactyly syndrome in twins: Beemer-Langer type with polydactyly. Clin Genet 50 : 159–163

Hennekam RCM (1991) Short rib syndrome – Beemer type in sibs. Am J Med Genet 40 : 230–233

Yang SS, Roth JA, Langer LO (1991) Short rib syndrome Beemer-Langer type with polydactyly: a multiple congenital anomalies syndrome. Am J Med Genet 39 : 243– 246

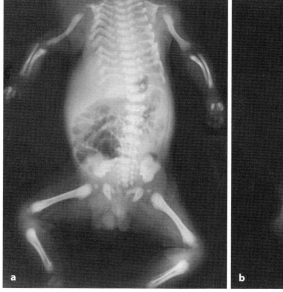
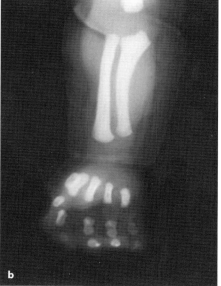

Fig. 3.36a, b. *Short rib (-polydactyly), Beemer-Langer type,* 38 weeks' gestation. **a** The chest is narrow due to shortened, horizontally oriented ribs. The ilia are well formed. Premature ossification centers of the capital femoral epiphyses are seen. The leg bones are mildly short but well modeled with round ends. The humeri, ulnae and radii are bowed. **b** Metacarpals and proximal phalanges are short but well formed; the middle and distal phalanges are small. Compare with hand bones in the Saldino-Noonan/Verma-Naumoff type of the short rib(-polydactyly) syndrome

Asphyxiating Thoracic Dysplasia   MIM 208500

Synonym: ATD; Jeune syndrome; asphyxiating thoracic dystrophy; thoracic-pelvic-phalangeal dystrophy.

Major Radiographic Features:

- Small thorax with short, often horizontally oriented ribs
- Small ilia bones with spur-like downward projection at the medial and lateral aspects of the acetabular roofs; premature ossification of the capital femoral ages
- Mildly shortened long tubular bones with round ends
- Short middle and distal phalanges
- Occasionally postaxial polydactyly

Mode of Inheritance: Autosomal recessive.

Prenatal Diagnosis: Sonography shows low thoracic circumference, increased nuchal translucency, sometimes short tubular bones. Hydrops may be present. The disorder has been detected at 14 weeks' gestation.

Differential Diagnosis: In the *Saldino-Noonan/Verma-Naumoff* and *Beemer-Langer* types of short-rib(-poly-dactyly) syndromes the tubular bones are more severely shortened. The *Majewski* type differs by the disproportionately short tibia. *Chondroectodermal dysplasia* differs by the more normal thorax and the presence of cardiac defects and gingival frenula. A narrow thorax may also be found in other bone dysplasias including *thanatophoric dysplasia* and *metatropic dysplasia*. These disorders are differentiated by the different spinal, pelvic, and long bone changes.

Prognosis: Neonatal mortality is increased due to cardiorespiratory compromise. With appropriate intensive care even severely affected infants may survive, become respiratory independent, and subsequently develop normally. Mildly affected patients have a good a priori prognosis.

Remarks: Patients with asphyxiating thoracic dysplasia and mild manifestations of short rib-(-polydactyly) type Saldino-Noonan/Verma-Naumoff have been observed in the same family (Ho et al. 1990), pointing to the possibility of a wide spectrum of disorders caused by allelic mutations of the same gene.

References

DenHollander NS, Robben SG, Hoogeboom AJ, Niermeijer MF, Wladimiroff JW (2001) Early prenatal sonographic diagnosis and follow-up of Jeune syndrome. Ultrasound Obstet Gynecol 18: 378–383

Ho NC et al (1990) Am J Med Genet 90:310

Kajantie E, Andersson S, Kaitila I (2001) Familial asphyxiating thoracic dysplasia: clinical variability and impact of improved neonatal intensive care. J Pediatr 139:130–133

Oberklaid F, Davies DM, Mayne V, Campbell P (1977) Asphyxiating thoracic dysplasia: clinical, radiological and pathological information on 10 Patients. Arch Dis Child 52:785–765

Schinzel A, Savoldelli G, Briner J, Schubiger G (1985) Prenatal sonographic diagnosis of Jeune syndrome. Radiology 154:777–778

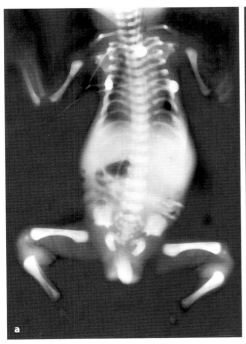
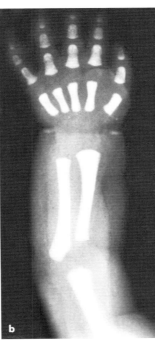

Fig. 3.37a, b. *Asphyxiating thoracic dysplasia.* **a** The ribs are short and the clavicles are elevated. The ilia are short in the vertical dimension with horizontal acetabular margins. Spurs of bone extend downward from the medial margins of the acetabula. The long tubular bones are mildly short and well modeled. **b** Radius and ulna are slightly short and thick. There is progressive proximal-distal shortening of the phalanges

Short Rib (-Polydactyly) Syndrome, Majewski Type   MIM 263520

Synonym: Short rib syndrome, Majewski type; Majewski syndrome; Short rib (-polydactyly) syndrome, type II; SRPS II.

Major Radiographic Features:

- Narrow chest with short, horizontally oriented ribs
- Normal pelvis
- Shortened tubular bones with smooth ends
- Tibia ovoid and shorter than fibula
- Pre- and/or postaxial polydactyly

Mode of Inheritance: Autosomal recessive.

Prenatal Diagnosis: Sonography shows narrow thorax and short tibiae. The fetus may be hydropic. Oligohydramnios has been observed in conjunction with glomerulocystic disease.

Differential Diagnosis: In the *Saldino-Noonan/Verma-Naumoff type* of short rib (-polydactyly) the metaphyseal margins are irregular and the fibulae are as short as the tibiae. In *asphyxiating thoracic dysplasia* and *Chondro-ectodermal dysp*lasia (Ellis-van Creveld syndrome) the tibiae are less severely shortened and the pelvis is abnormal with characteristic spurs.

Prognosis: The patients die shortly after birth from cardiorespiratory insufficiency.

Remarks: The Majewski syndrome may be part of a continuous spectrum of disorders that includes patients with the oro-facio-digital syndromes II and IV. Short tibiae, but not short ribs have been observed in the oro-facio-digital syndromes. Disproportionately short tibiae have also been described in an X-linked recessive condition without short ribs but otherwise resembling the oro-facio-digital syndrome II (Edwards et al. 1988).

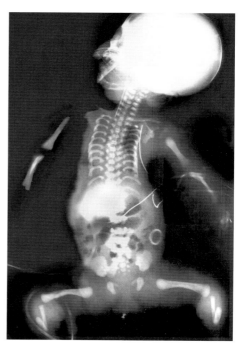

Fig. 3.38. *Short rib- (polydactyly) syndrome, Majewski type.* The ribs are short and horizontal. The pelvic appearance is normal. The tibiae are considerably shorter than the fibulae and their contours are rounded

References

Edwards M et al (1988) Clin Genet 34:325

Meinecke P, Hazek H (1990) Orofaciodigital syndrome type IV (Mohr-Majewski syndrome) with severe expression expanding the known spectrum of anomalies. J Med Genet 27:200–202

Montemarano H, Bulas DI, Chyandra R, Tifft C (1995) Prenatal diagnosis of glomerulocystic kidney disease in short-rib polydactyly syndrome type II, Majewski type. Pediatr Radiol 235:469–471

Spranger JW, Brill PWE, Poznanski A (2002) Bone dysplasias, 2nd edn. Urban-Fischer, Oxford

Ellis-van Creveld Syndrome MIM 255500

Synonym: EvC; Chondroectodermal dysplasia; Mesoectodermal dysplasia.

Major Radiographic Features:
- Pelvic dysplasia with low ilia; hook-like downward protrusion of the medial and frequently also of the lateral aspects of the acetabulum; often premature ossification of the capital femoral epiphyses
- Mild shortness of the long tubular bones
- Progressive proximal-distal shortening of the tubular bones of hands and feet; polydactyly
- Sometimes narrow thorax

Mode of Inheritance: Autosomal recessive.

Molecular Basis: The Ellis-van Creveld syndrome is caused by mutations of either the *EvC* gene or the *EvC2* gene, both located in the same region on chromosome 4p16. The function of these genes is still unknown.

Prenatal Diagnosis: Short limbs, polydactyly, narrow thorax, and ventricular septal defect have been prenatally recognized by ultrasound.

Differential Diagnosis: *Asphyxiating thoracic dysplasia* (ATD) closely resembles the Ellis-van Creveld syndrome (EvC). The ribs are usually shorter in ATD and polydactyly is less common. Heart defects and gingival frenula are characteristics of EvC but not of ATD. In *short rib (-polydactyly), Majewski type* the pelvic appearance is normal and the tibia is shorter than the fibula.

Prognosis: Infantile mortality is elevated due to pulmonary and cardiac complications. However, most patients survive and their further prognosis *quo ad vitam* is good.

Remarks: Heterozygous parents may be asymptotic or have dental anomalies, postaxial polydactyly, and nail dysplasia (Weyers syndrome). Like the Majewski type of short rib (-polydactyly), the Ellis-van Creveld syndrome is part of the orofacial-digital spectrum of disorders. The phenotypic similarity of asphyxiating thoracic dysplasia and the Ellis-van Creveld syndrome points to common pathogenic mechanisms.

References

Dugoff L, Thieme G, Hobbins (2001) First trimester prenatal diagnosis of chondroectodermal dysplasia (Ellis-van Creveld syndrome) with ultrasound. Ultrasound Obstet Gynecol 17:86–88

McKusick Va, Egeland JA, Eldridge R, Krusen DE (1964) Dwarfism in the Amish. I. The Ellis-van Creveld syndrome. Bull Johns Hopkins Hosp 115:306–333

Parilla BV, Leeth EA, Kambich MP, Chilis P, MacGregor SN (2003) J Ultrasound Med 255–258

Riuz-Perez VL, Tompson SWJ, Blair HJ et al (2003) Mutations in two nonhomologous genes in a head-to-head configuration cause Ellis-van Creveld syndrome. Am J Hum Genet 72:728–732

Sergi C, Voiglander T, Zoubaa S et al (2001) Ellis-van Creveld syndrome: a generalized dysplasia of enchondral ossification. Pediatr Radiol 189–193

Spranger S, Tariverdian G (1995) Symptomatic heterozygosity in the Ellis-van Creveld syndrome. Clin Genet 47:217–220

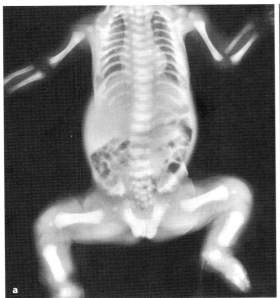
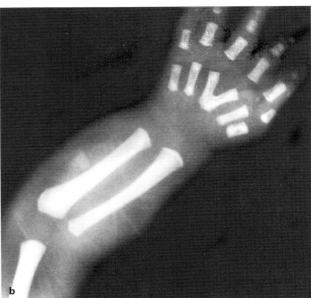

Fig. 3.39a, b. *Ellis van Creveld syndrome.* **a** The ribs are slightly short. The ilia are vertically short, and their inferior margins are horizontal with a downward-pointing hook at their medial ends. Femora and tibiae are short and broad. There is premature ossification of the capital femoral epiphyses. **b** The proximal end of the ulna and the distal end of the radius are wide; both bones are shorter than normal. An intercalary hexadactyly and proximal-distal shortening of the tubular bones of the hands are noted

Greenberg Dysplasia   MIM 215140

Synonyms: Hydrops-ectopic calcification – moth-eaten skeletal dysplasia; HEM/Greenberg skeletal dysplasia; includes dappled-diaphysis dysplasia.

Major Radiographic Features:
- Defective ossification of the calvaria
- Disruption of the facial bones and the axial and appendicular skeletons into small islands of ossification

Mode of Inheritance: Autosomal recessive.

Molecular Basis: Mutations of the *LMB* gene on chromosome 1q42.1 encoding Lamin B receptor, a sterol delta(14)-reductase that interferes with cholesterol biosynthesis, as demonstrated by elevated levels of cholesta-8,14-dien-3beta-ol in cultured fibroblasts.

Prenatal Diagnosis: Fetal sonography in the second trimester shows hydrops fetalis, severe micromelia, and irregular hyperechogenic foci in the ribs and long bones.

Differential Diagnosis: *X-linked dominant chondrodysplasia punctata* differs by the asymmetric, scattered appearance of punctate calcifications. In *autosomal recessive chondrodysplasia punctata*, the vertebral bodies are better ossified and the tubular bones are not as severely disrupted as in Greenberg dysplasia.

Prognosis: The fetuses are hydropic and in none of the published cases have survived to the end of gestation.

Remarks: In a disorder called dappled diaphysis dysplasia the shafts of the tubular bones are even more severely fragmented than in some cases of Greenberg dysplasia (Carty et al. 1989). The two disorders are most probably allelic.

References

Carty et al (1989) Fortschr Rontgenstr 150:228

Greenberg CR, Rimoin DL, Gruber H, DeSa DJB, Reed M, Lachman RS (1988) A new autosomal recessive lethal chondrodystrophy with congenital hydrops. Am J Med Genet 29:623–632

Horn LC, Faber R, Meiner A, Piskazeck U, Spranger J (2000) Greenberg dysplasia: first reported case with additional non-skeletal malformations and without consanguinity Prenat Diagn 20:1008–1011

Madazli R, Aksoy, F, Ocak V, Atasü T (2001) Detailed ultrasonographic findings in Greenberg dysplasia. Prenatal Diagn 21:65–67

Waterham HR, Koster J, Moozer P et al (2003) Autosomal recessive HEM/Greenberg skeletal dysplasia is caused by 3-β-hydroxysterol Δ^{14} reductase deficiency due to mutations in the lamin B receptor gene. Am J Hum Genet 72:1013–1017

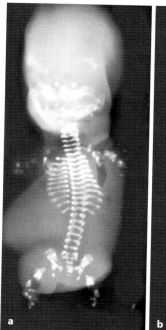
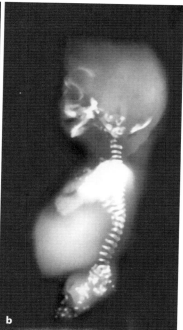

Fig. 3.40a, b. *Greenberg dysplasia.* The calvarium is unossified. The rest of the skeleton, with the exception of the irregularly ossified ribs and vertebral arches, is disrupted into a multitude of radiodensities. The contours of the flattened vertebral bodies are still discernible

Chondrodysplasia Punctata, X-Linked Dominant   MIM 302960

Synonym: Conradi-Hünermann syndrome; Conradi-Hünermann-Happle syndrome, Happle syndrome, CdpXL.

Major Radiographic Features:
- Punctate calcifications mostly of long bone ends, carpal and tarsal regions, spinous and transverse processes, sometimes laryngeal cartilage
- Irregular shapes of the vertebral bodies
- Sometimes asymmetric shortness of the long bones

Mode of Inheritance: X-linked dominant, lethal in hemizygous males.

Molecular Basis: Mutations in the *EBP* (emopamil) gene located on Xp11.23-p11.22 encoding β-hydroxysteroid Δ^8, Δ^7 -isomerase responsible for typical and atypical forms of X-linked dominant chondrodysplasia punctata, including some cases with the CHILD syndrome.

Prenatal Diagnosis: Sonography in the 2nd trimester has revealed asymmetric limb shortening.

Differential Diagnosis: In *autosomal recessive (rhizomelic) chondrodysplasia punctata* marked shortness of the humeri and femora and coronal clefts are noted. The CHILD syndrome is characterized by unilateral ichthyosiform erythroderma with ipsilateral limb defects and stippling (Fig. 3.42). *X-linked chromosomal-recessive chondrodysplasia punctata* is differentiated by the presence of exquisitely short distal phalanges (Fig. 3.43).

Prognosis: With few exceptions the disorder is lethal in males. Most affected females survive the neonatal period and develop normally except for localized growth disturbance in stippled bone areas, ichthyosiform skin changes, and partial alopecia.

Remarks: Punctate calcifications are nonspecific and occur in numerous conditions including the Zellweger syndrome; the Smith-Lemli-Opitz syndrome; mucolipidosis II after exposure to warfarin, anticonvulsants, and alcohol; and in maternal vitamin K deficiency. Congenital hemidysplasia with ichthyosiform erythroderma and limb defects (CHILD syndrome; Fig. 3.42) is genetically heterogeneous and can also be caused by mutations of the *NSDHL* gene at Xq28. Chondrodysplasia punctata, tibia-metacarpal type, is the term used for a phenotype with prominent involvement of the tibiae and metacarpals.

References

Happle R (1979) X-linked dominant chondrodysplasia punctata: review of the literature and report of a case. Hum Genet 53:65–73

Happle R, Koch H, Lenz W (1980) The CHILD syndrome: congenital hemidysplasia with ichthyosiform erythroderma and limb defects. Eur J Pediatr 134:27–33

Ikegawa S, Ohashi H, Ogata T et al (2000) Novel and recurrent EBP mutations in X-linked dominant chondrodysplasia punctata. Am J Med Genet 94:300–305

Pradhan GM, Chaub al NG, Chaubal HN, Raghavan J (2002) Second-trimester sonographic diagnosis of nonrhizomelic chondrodysplasia punctata. J Ultrasound Med 21:345–349

Spranger JW, Brill, PW, Poznanski A (2002) Bone dysplasias, 2nd edn. Urban/Fischer/Oxford Press, Munich

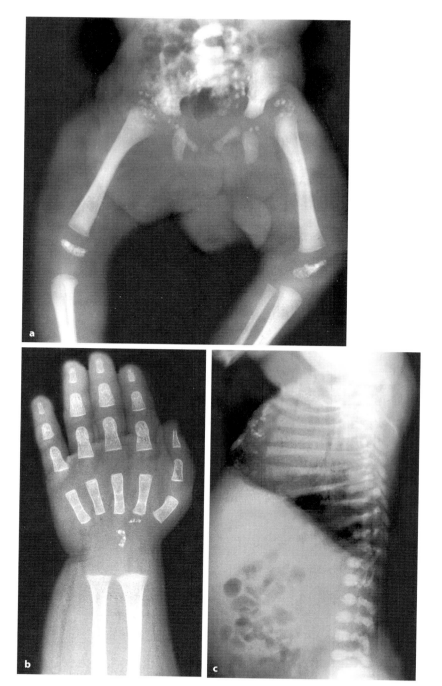

Fig. 3.41a–c. *Chondrodysplasia punctata X-linked dominant.* **a, b** Punctate calcifications are seen in the pelvis, in the proximal epiphyses of the femora, the knees and the carpal bones. **c** The form of the vertebral bodies is slightly irregular. There are puncta in the sternum and in the arches of the upper lumbar vertebrae

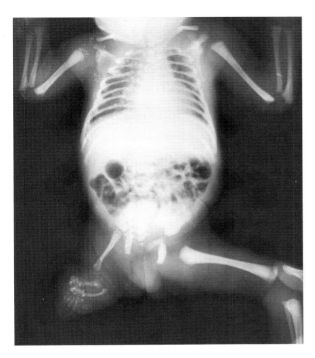

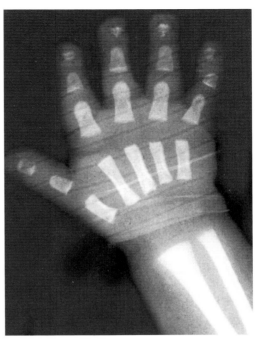

Fig. 3.42. *CHILD syndrome.* The bones of the right leg are small and misshapen. Extensive punctate calcifications are present in the right foot. The rest of the skeleton is normal

Fig. 3.43. *X-linked recessive chondrodysplasia punctata* (brachytele-phalangic type of chondrodysplasia punctata). The distal phalanges are short and irregularly ossified

Chondrodysplasia Punctata, Rhizomelic Type   MIM 215100

Synonyms: Rhizomelic chondrodysplasia punctata; autosomal recessive chondrodysplasia punctata; RCDP.

Major Radiographic Features:

- Coronal clefts composed of cartilage separating anterior and posterior ossification centers of vertebral bodies, which clefts are best seen in infancy and may no longer be apparent in the older child as the cartilage ossifies
- Very short humeri and relatively short femora with some metaphyseal splaying
- Punctate epiphyses at the ends of the long bones which disappear after 1–3 years

Genetic Transmission:
Autosomal recessive; genetic heterogeneity (see molecular pathology).

Molecular Basis:

- RCDP, type 1: Mutation in the *PEX7* gene located at 6q22-q24 encoding the receptor for peroxisomal matrix proteins with the type 2 peroxisome targeting signal, which defect interferes with peroxisome biogenesis and leads to multiple defects in peroxisome function.
- RCDP, type 2: Mutation of the *DHAPAT* gene located on chromosome 1 encoding the peroxisomal enzyme acyl-CoA: dihydroxyacetonephosphate acyltransferase, an enzyme essential for the formation of ether phospholipids.
- RCDP, type 3: Mutations in the *AGPS* gene located on 2q31 encoding alkyldihydroxyacetone phosphate (DHAP) synthase required for a single step in the biosynthesis for plasmalogens.

Prenatal Diagnosis:
Severe rhizomelic limb shortening, premature ossification and stippling of multiple epiphyses have been detected by fetal sonography. Knowledge of the specific mutation from a previously affected child will allow for molecular analysis in chorionic villi.

Prognosis:
The prognosis is poor. Affected infants fail to thrive, are severely retarded in their psychomotor development, and usually die in infancy from repeated infections. Some survive into childhood; the oldest reported lived to 16 years. Survivors have severe psychomotor retardation, spastic tetraplegia, and thermoregulatory instability.

Major Differential Diagnoses:
The asymmetric distribution of punctate calcifications and irregular abnormalities of the vertebral bodies differentiate *X-linked dominant chondrodysplasia punctata* from the rhizomelic type. The *Zellweger syndrome*, also a peroxisomal disorder, has puncta in the patellar area and usually does not have coronal clefts. Isolated puncta occur in *many acquired and genetic conditions* and frequently involve only the tarsal bones.

Remarks:
The various types of RCDP cannot be differentiated on clinical or radiographic grounds; their differentiation requires biochemical or molecular analysis. RCDP type 1 is by far the most common type. Varying severity of clinical manifestations within type 1 RCDP is explained by allelic mutations leading to varying residual activity of the mutant protein.

References

Braverman N, Chen L, Obie C, Moser A et al (2002) Mutation analysis of PEX 7 in 60 probands with rhizomelic chondrodysplasia punctata and functional correlations of genotype with phenotype. Hum Mutat 20:284–287

Gilbert EF, Opitz JM, Spranger JW, Langer JR LO, Wolfson JJ, Visekul C (1976) Chondrodysplasia Punctata-Rhizomelic form: pathologic and radiologic studies of three infants. Eur J Pediatr 12:89–109

Hertzberg BS, Kliewer MA, Decker M, Miller CR, Bowie JD (1999) Antenatal ultrasonographic diagnosis of rhizomelic chondrodysplasia punctata. J Ultrasound Med 18:715–718

Wardinsky TD, Pagon RA, Powell BR, Mcgillivray B, Stephan M, Zonana J, Moser A (1990) rhizomelic chondrodysplasia punctata and survival beyond one year: a review of the literature and five case reports. Clin Genet 38:84–93

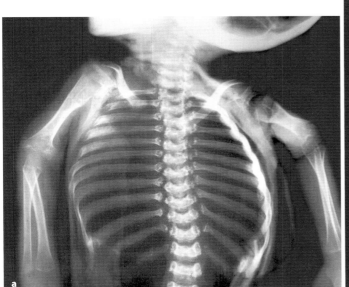
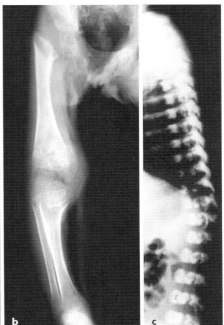

Fig. 3.44a–c. *Chondrodysplasia punctata, rhizomelic type.* **a, b** The humeri and femora are short with a "sawed-off" appearance of their ends. The ribs are broad with irregularly calcified proximal ends. There is less marked shortness of the tibia. Note the normal appearance of the bones of the forearm. Areas of irregular calcification are not seen in this patient but may be present in others. **c** There are coronal clefts in the lumbar vertebral bodies

Larsen Syndrome   MIM 150250, 245600, 245650

Major Radiographic Features:

- Multiple dislocations, most notably in the hips, knees, and elbows
- Often disproportionately large cranium
- Occasionally hypoplasia of the distal humerus

Mode of Inheritance: It is autosomal dominant in most cases. The condition has been observed in multiple children of unaffected parents. This may be due to non-penetrance in an affected parent, germinal parental mosaicism, or true genetic heterogeneity. The autosomal recessive Réunion form of the Larsen syndrome is characterized by very short stature and the frequent presence of radio-ulnar synostosis.

Molecular Basis: Mutations of the FNLB gene located on 3p14.3 enoding filamin B, a protein regulating the organization of the cytoskeletal F-actin.

Prenatal Diagnosis: The disorder has been detected prenatally by ultrasound showing abnormal position of the knee joints and clubfeet. However, abnormally positioned limbs in a fetus are nonspecific and do not allow a diagnosis of Larsen syndrome.

Differential Diagnosis: Hypoplastic distal humeri are seen in *Omodysplasia*, which differs by the associated distal femoral hypoplasia and absence of dislocated hips. The *Desbuquois syndrome* is differentiated by the presence of coronal clefts of the vertebral bodies and the abnormal position and form of finger bones, if present.

Dislocated hips and elbows sometimes occur in the *oto-palatodigital syndrome I*. Differentiation is possible by molecular analysis showing a mutated *FNLA* gene in OPD.

Prognosis: Most patients survive to adulthood. Early death due to pulmonary hypoplasia has been reported.

Remarks: Manifestations of the Larsen syndrome are highly variable; differentiation of the Larsen syndrome from other disorders with multiple congenital dislocations, notably oto-palato-digital syndrome, may be difficult at birth.

References

Alembick Y, Stoll C, Messer J (1997) On the phenotypic overlap between "severe" oto-palato-digital type II syndrome and Larsen syndrome. Variable manifestation of a single autosomal dominant gene. Genet Couns 8:133–137

Becker R, Wegner RD, Kunze J (2000) Clinical variability of Larsen syndrome: diagnosis in a father after sonographic detection of a severely affected fetus. Clin Genet 57:148–150

Krakow D, Robertson SP, King LM et al. (2004) Mutations in the gene encoding filamin B disrupt vertebral segmentation, joint formation and skeletogenesis. Nature Genet Adv Online Pub, Feb 29

Latta LJ, Graham JB, Aase JM, Scham SM, Smith DW (1981) Larsen syndrome: a skeletal dysplasia with multiple joint dislocations and unusual facies. J Pediatr 78:291–298

Mortello D, Hoechstetter L, Bendon RW, Dignan PSJ, Oestreich AD, Siddiqi J (1991) Prenatal diagnosis of recurrent Larsen syndrome: further definition of a lethal variant. Prenat Diagn 11:215–225

Spranger JW, Brill PWE, Poznanski A (2002) Bone dysplasia, 2nd edn., Elsevier GmbH, Urban & Fischer, Munich

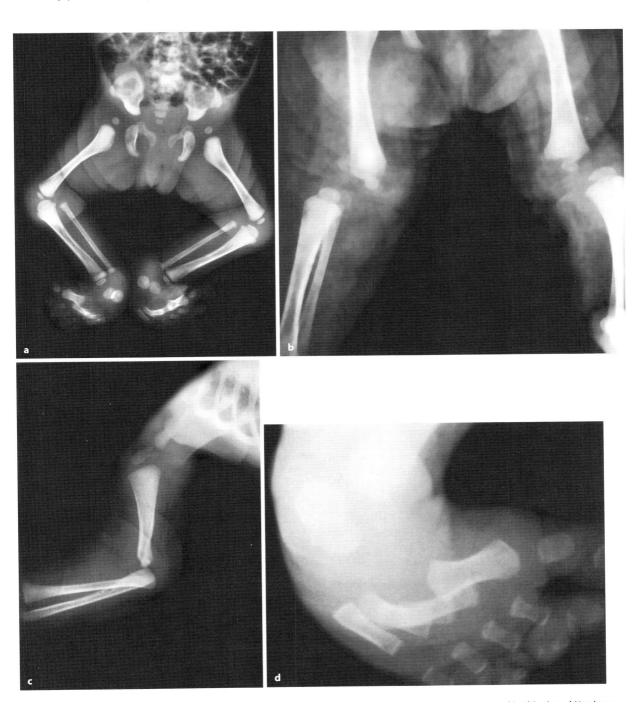

Fig. 3.45a–d. *Larsen syndrome.* **a** Three months. The acetabular fossae are underdeveloped due to congenitally dislocated hips. **b** Newborn. Both knees are dislocated anteriorly and laterally. **c** Newborn. The humerus is short and distally tapered. Lateral dislocation of the radial head is not demonstrated in this view. **d** Newborn. There is a marked equinovarus deformity of the foot. (From: Spranger et al.: Bone Dysplasias, 2nd edn., 2002, with kind permission from Elsevier GmbH, Urban & Fischer, Munich)

Desbuquois Dysplasia   MIM 251450

Synonym: Micromelic dwarfism with vertebral and metaphyseal abnormalities and advanced carpotarsal ossification.

Major Radiographic Features:
- Coronal clefts of vertebral bodies
- Hypoplastic lower ilia
- Short femoral necks
- Dislocated hips and knees in severe cases
- Advanced carpotarsal ossification
- Often short first metacarpal bone
- Often extra ossicles between metacarpals and proximal phalanges of the first and second fingers

Mode of Inheritance: Autosomal recessive.

Molecular Basis: Causative gene mapped to chromosome 17q25.3.

Prenatal Diagnosis: Prenatal diagnosis has to this date not been reported, but should be possible on the basis of short limbs and abnormal limb posture in severely affected patients.

Differential Diagnosis: In the *Larsen syndrome*, dislocated joints and coronal clefts of the vertebral bodies are more prominent. Severe cases of the *oto-palato-digital syndrome* show more irregular, bowed long tubular bones. Molecular analysis shows a mutated *FNLA* gene in X-linked OPD but not in the autosomal recessive Desbuquois syndrome. Hand changes similar to those in the Desbuquois syndrome are seen in the *Catel-Manzke syndrome,* which differs by the absence of other skeletal defects.

Prognosis: Neonatal and early infantile mortality is increased due to respiratory failure, but more than 70% of the patients survive.

Remarks: The clinical and radiological manifestations of the Desbuquois syndrome are variable and range from mild joint laxity with almost normal hand bones to multiple congenital dislocations and ossicles of fingers and toes. A. congenital, autosomal recessive multiple dislocation syndrome seen on Réunion Island (MIM 245600) may be identical or pathogenetically related to the Desbuquois syndrome.

References

Faivre L, Le Merrer M, Al-Gazali LI, Ausems MGEM, Bitoun P, Bacq P, Maroteaux P, Munnich A, Cormier-Daire V (2003) Homozygosity mapping of a Desbuquois dysplasia locus to chromosome 17q25.3. J Med Genet 40:282–284

Hall BE (2001) Lethality in Desbuquois dysplasia: three new cases. Pediatr Radiol 31:43–47

Shohat M, Lachman R, Gruber ED, Hsia YE, Golbus MS, Wiss DR, Bodell A, Bryke ER, Hogge WA, Rimoin D (1994) Desbuquois syndrome: clinical, radiographic, and morphologic characterization. Am J Med Genet 52:9–18

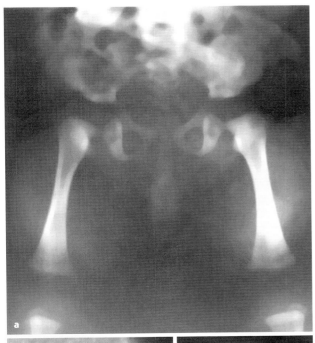

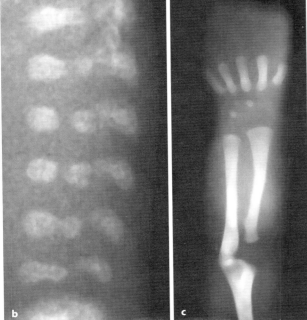

Fig. 3.46a–c. *Desbuquois syndrome, full-term newborn.*
a The vertical dimension of the ilia is decreased and the femoral necks are short with a slight prominence of the lesser trochanter producing the appearance of a monkey wrench. The femora are short. **b** The vertebral bodies are flattened with distinct coronal clefts. **c** Carpal ossification in this newborn is grossly advanced

Atelosteogenesis   MIM 112310, 108720, 109721

Synonym: Includes Boomerang dysplasia, Piepkorn type of lethal osteochondrodysplasia, Atelosteogenesis I, Atelosteogenesis III.

Major Radiographic Features:
- Shortened, misshapen, in severe cases unossified long tubular bones
- Short, misshapen, in severe cases unossified tubular bones of the hands and feet
- Coronal clefts of the vertebral bodies and in severe cases unossified vertebral bodies

Mode of Inheritance: Autosomal dominant.

Molecular Basis: Mutations of the FNLB gene located on 3p14.3 enoding filamin B, a protein regulating the organization of the cytoskeletal F-actin.

Prenatal Diagnosis: Short, partially unossified tubular bones are detected by sonography. Polyhydramnios is commonly present.

Differential Diagnosis: Mild cases of atelosteogenesis resemble *severe diastrophic dysplasia* (*De la Chapelle dysplasia*), which differs by the preserved metaphyseal flare, irregular diaphyseal contours of the long tubular bones, and mutated *DTDST* gene. "Absent bones" due to widespread lack of ossification are noted in severe *hypophosphatasia*. In that disorder poor ossification involves the ribs, which are well preserved in atelosteogenesis, and grossly deformed tubular bones are not seen.

Prognosis: Patients with severe atelosteogenesis are stillborn or die shortly after birth. Patients with mild (type III) atelosteogenesis may survive into adulthood.

Remarks: Boomerang dysplasia, Atelosteogenesis I, III and the Larsen syndrome are caused by defects of filamin A forming a continuous spectrum of disorders. The phenotypic overlap of these conditions with the Oto-palatodigital family of disorders expresses their common pathogenesis, genetically determined errors of the cytoskeleton.

References
Beijani BA, Oberg K, Wilkins I, Moise A, Langston C, Superti-Furga A, Lupski JR (1998) Prenatal ultrasonographic description and postnatal pathological findings in atelosteogenesis type 1. Am J Med Genet 79 : 392–395

Krakow D, Robertson SP, King LM et al. (2004) Mutations in the gene encoding filamin B disrupt vertebral segmentation, joint formation and skeletogenesis. Nature Genet Adv Online Pub, Feb 29

Nishimura G, Horiuchi T, Kim OH, Sasamoto Y (1997) Atypical skeletal changes in otopalatodigital syndrome type II: Phenotypic overlap among otopalatodigital syndrome type II, Boomerang dysplasia, Atelosteogenesis type I and type III, and lethal male phenotype of Melnick-Needles Syndrome. Am J Med Genet 73 : 132–138

Odent S, Loget P, Le Marec B, Delezoide AL, Maroteaux P (1999) Unusual fan shaped ossification in a female fetus with radiological features of boomerang dysplasia. J Pediatr Radiol 26 : 678–679

Schultz C, Langer LO, Laxova R, Pauli RM (1999) Atelosteogenesis type III: long term survival, prenatal diagnosis, and evidence for dominant transmission. Am J Med Genet 83 : 28–42

Sillence D, Worthington S, Dixon J, Osborn R, Kozlowski KL (1997) Atelosteogenesis syndromes: a review, with comments on their pathogenesis. Pediatr Radiol 27 : 388–396

Spranger JW, Brill PWE, Poznanski A (2002) Bone dysplasia, 2nd edn., Elsevier GmbH, Urban & Fischer, Munich

Ueno K, Tanaka M, Mizakoshi K, Zhao C, Shinmoto H, Nishimura G, Yoshimaro Y (2002) Prenatal diagnosis of atelosteogenesis I at 21 weeks' gestation. Prenat Diagn 22 : 1071–1075

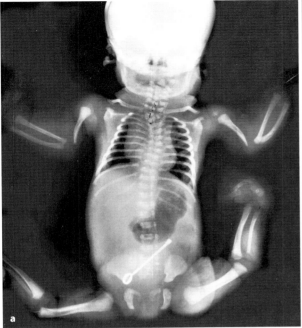
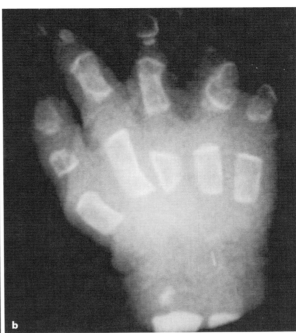

Fig. 3.47. a *Atelosteogenesis III.* Ossification of the vertebrae at the cervico-thoracic junction is irregular. The distal humeri are hypoplastic. The basilar portions of the ilia are narrow and the distal portions of the femora are mildly hypoplastic. **b** The metacarpal bones and phalanges are variably short, squared and misshapen. There is an irregular ossification center at the distal radius. (From: Spranger et al.: Bone Dysplasias, 2nd edn., 2002, with kind permission from Elsevier GmbH, Urban & Fischer, Munich)

De la Chapelle Dysplasia   MIM 256050

Synonym: Atelosteogenesis II.

Major Radiographic Features:
- Shortened tubular bones with flared ends
- Distal tapering of humeri
- Shortened, sometimes triangular ulna and fibula; less severely shortened, bowed radius and tibia
- Shortened, misshapen tubular bones of the hands and feet; globular appearance of metacarpal I and metatarsal I

Mode of Inheritance: Autosomal recessive.

Molecular Basis: Mutations of the diastrophic dysplasia sulfate transporter gene *DTDST*.

Prenatal Diagnosis: Short limbs have been detected by ultrasound at 21 weeks of gestation. In familial cases prenatal diagnosis may be achieved by molecular analysis.

Differential Diagnosis: The tubular bones in *atelosteogenesis I/III* show less metaphyseal flare and the tubular bones of the hands are more plump. In *achondrogenesis IB* ossification of the spine and limbs is more defective. Irregular, short tubular bones and a rounded metacarpal I are found in *diastrophic dysplasia,* which differs by the more normal appearing long tubular bones.

Prognosis: Most patients are stillborn or die shortly after birth. There is overlap with diastrophic dysplasia which has a good prognosis.

Remarks: The clinical spectrum of *DTDST* mutations encompasses achondrogenesis IB, De la Chapelle dysplasia, diastrophic dysplasia, and a relatively mild, late-manifesting form of multiple epiphyseal dysplasia. In spite of their common molecular basis, these disorders are listed as separate diseases because of their different clinical manifestations and course. The name atelosteogenesis II had been chosen because of the phenotypic similarity with atelosteogenesis I/III, which, however, seems to have a different molecular basis.

References

Hästbacka J, Superti-Furga A, Wilcox WR, Rimoin DL, Cohn DH, Lander ES (1996) Atelosteogenesis type II is caused by mutations in the diastrophic dysplasia sulfate-transporter gene (DTDST): evidence for a phenotypic series involving three chondrodysplasias. Am J HumAGement 58:255–262

Nores JA, Rotmensch S, Romero R, Avila C, Inati M, Hobbins JC (1992) Atelosteogenesis type II: sonographic and radiological correlation. Prenat Diagn 12:741–753

Sillence DO, Kozlowski K, Rogers JG, Sprague PL, Cullitz GJ, Osborn RA (1987) Atelosteogenesis: evidence for heterogeneity. Pediatr Radiol 12:112–118

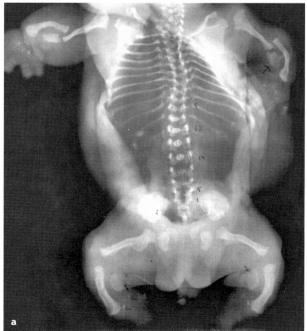

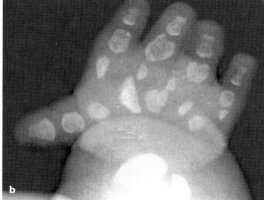

Fig. 3.48a, b. *De la Chapelle dysplasia.* **a** At 38 weeks' gestation. The upper thorax is narrow with overconstriction of the midthoracic vertebrae Note distal tapering of the humeri, very short, triangular ulnae, and relatively long, bowed radii. Metacarpals and phalanges are seen as small, irregular bone islands. Femora and tibiae are bowed with wide ends. The fibulae are very short and halberd shaped. **b** At 40 weeks' gestation. Metacarpals and phalanges are grossly irregular in size and shape with an extra bone in the basis of the third digit

Diastrophic Dysplasia   MIM 222600

Major Radiographic Features:
- Shortened tubular bones with wide ends
- Disproportionate shortness of the first metacarpal
- Club feet

Mode of Inheritance: Autosomal recessive.

Molecular Basis: Mutations of the *DTDST* gene located on chromosome impede the function of a transmembrane protein that transports sulfate into chondrocytes. Lack of intracellular sulfate results in undersulfated proteoglycans.

Prenatal Diagnosis: Short limbs and short, abducted thumbs and great toes have been detected at 20 weeks' gestation by ultrasound. By transvaginal sonography the diagnosis has been suspected at 13 weeks' gestation. If the mutation is known, molecular analysis should be possible in chorionic tissue and cultured amnion cells.

Differential Diagnosis: The long bone changes of diastrophic dysplasia are much milder than those in *de la Chapelle dysplasia* and *achondrogenesis IB*. The vertebral bodies are normal in diastrophic dysplasia. *Omodysplasia* is differentiated by distal hypoplasia of the humeri and femora as well as the normal hand bones.

Prognosis: Perinatal and early infant mortality is increased, but once stabilized, the infants grow up with a normal life expectancy.

Remarks: Achondrogenesis I B, de la Chapelle dysplasia, diastrophic dysplasia, and autosomal recessive epiphyseal dysplasia are members of an etiopathogenic family caused by allelic mutations of the *DTDST* gene. More severe phenotypes result from a more defective sulfate transport and mild phenotypes from partial defects.

References
Langer LO (1965) Diastrophic dwarfism in early infancy. Am J Roentgenol 93:399–304

Karniski LP (2001) Mutations in the diastrophic dysplasia sulfate transporter (DTDST) gene: correlation between sulfate transport activity and chondrodysplasia phenotype. Hum Mol Genet 10:1485–1490

Rossi A, Superti-Furga A (2001) Mutations in the diastrophic dysplasia sulfate transporter (DTDST) gene (SLC26A2): 22 novel mutations, mutation review, associated skeletal phenotypes, and diagnostic relevance. Hum Mutat 17:159–171

Severi FM, Bocchi C, Sanseverino F, Petraglia F (2003) Prenatal ultrasonographic diagnosis of diastrophic dysplasia at 13 weeks of gestation. J Matern Fetal Neonatal Med 13:282–284

Tongsong T, Wanapirak C, Sirichotiyakul S, Chanprapaph P (2002) Prenatal sonographic diagnosis of diastrophic dwarfism. J Clin Ultrasound 30:103–195

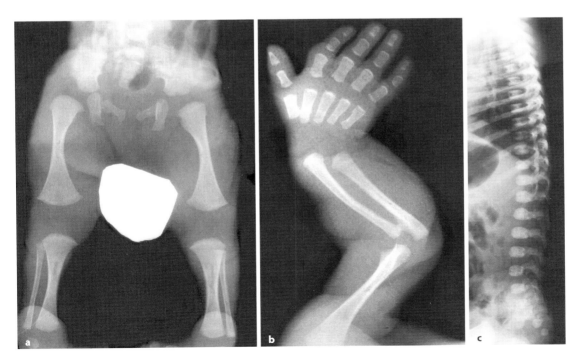

Fig. 3.49a–c. *Diastrophic dysplasia.* Newborn, 38 weeks' gestation. **a** The tubular bones are short with wide metaphyses. The knee epiphyses are not ossified. **b** The distal humerus is slightly tapered. The phalanges are short and squared. **c** A lateral spine film shows no major abnormalities

Omodysplasia   MIM 258315, 251455, 268250

Major Radiographic Features:
- Shortened arm and leg bones
- Club-shaped, distally tapered humerus and femur
- Dislocated radial heads
- Short first metacarpal in autosomal dominant cases

Mode of Inheritance: Omodysplasia is heterogeneous. Autosomal dominant inheritance has been found in slightly milder cases, autosomal recessive inheritance in more severe cases.

Prenatal Diagnosis: Short arms and legs have been detected by sonography at 17 weeks' gestation.

Differential Diagnosis: A short first metacarpal may be seen in *diastrophic dysplasia*, which differs by the absent club shape of humerus and femur and by the presence of club feet. Distally tapered humeri and femora are found in *atelosteogenesis*, which differs by the characteristic abnormalities of the bones of the hands and feet. Mesomelic dysplasia in *Robinow syndrome* is not associated with the humero-femoral abnormalities characterizing omodysplasia.

Prognosis: Except for physical shortness and restricted mobility of the elbows, development is normal.

Remarks: Marked phenotypic overlap between the dominant and recessive forms of omodysplasia suggests common pathogenetic mechanisms. The genetic and pathophysiologic relationship between omodysplasia and the Robinow syndrome remains to be established.

References

Borochowitz Z, Sabo E, Misselevitch I, Boss JH (1998) Autosomal-recessive omodysplasia: Prenatal diagnosis and histomorphometric assessment of the epiphyseal plates of the long bones. Am J Med Genet 76:238–244

Maroteaux P, Sauvegrain J, Chrispin A, Farriaux JP (1989) Omodysplasia. Am J Med Genet 32:371–375

Masel JP, Kozlowski K, Kiss P (1998) Autosomal recessive omodysplasia: report of three additional cases. Pediatr Radiol 28:608–611

Venditti CP, Farmer J, Russell KL et al (2002) Omodysplasia: an affected mother and son. Am J Med Genet 111:169–177

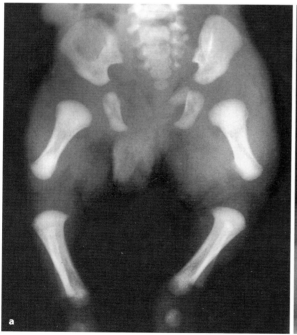
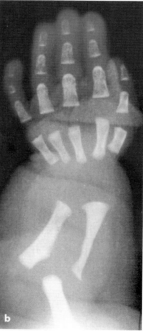

Fig. 3.50a, b. *Omodysplasia, autosomal recessive.* Newborn. **a** The femora are short with rounded, proximally wide and distally tapered ends producing a club-like appearance. The tibiae and fibulae are short. **b** Note short radius and ulna with dislocated radius. In this patient with recessive omodysplasia the hand bones are normal

Cleidocranial Dysplasia   MIM 119600

Synonym: Cleidocranial dysostosis; Pelvico-cleido-cranial dysostosis; cleido-cranio-digital dysostosis; osteo-dental dysplasia; Marie-Sainton disease; Scheuthauer-Marie-Sainton syndrome.

Major Radiographic Features:
- Retarded ossification of the calvaria and skull base
- Partial or total, uni-or bilateral absence of the clavicles
- Absent ossification of the pubic bones
- Short distal phalanges
- In severe cases, decreased mineralization with mild bowing of lower limbs

Mode of Inheritance: Autosomal dominant.

Molecular Basis: Mutations of the transcription factor *CBFA1* on chromosome 6p21.

Prenatal Diagnosis: Cleidocranial dysplasia has been diagnosed at 14 weeks' gestation on the basis of hypoplastic clavicles and underossified skull bones. In familial cases, molecular analysis should be attempted.

Differential Diagnosis: Abnormal clavicles are present in numerous conditions, which are differentiated by analysis of the rest of the skeleton. No other skeletal abnormalities are present in *congenital pseudarthrosis* of the clavicle. *Pyknodysostosis* differs by the increased bone density. The *Yunis-Varon syndrome* is characterized by the presence of distal reduction defects, notably a/hypoplasia of thumbs and great toes. The *Crane-Heise syndrome* is differentiated by cleft palate, micrognathia, and defective ossification of cervical vertebral bodies. Hypoplastic clavicles have also be reported in *cytogenetic abnormalities* including duplication of chromosome 8p22, partial trisomy 11q, partial trisomy 11q/22q, and trisomy 20p.

Prognosis: Life expectancy and mental development are normal. Dental, auditory, and respiratory problems may require medical attention in later life.

Remarks: Phenotypic variability is caused by allelic mutations of the *CBFA1* gene that result in a spectrum extending from severe, to classic, to mild manifestations, to isolated primary dental anomalies. Parental mosaicism may result in mild somatic manifestations and may be responsible for the rare occurrence of the disorder in children of unaffected parents.

References

Cooper SC, Flaitz CM, Johnston DA, Lee B, Hecht JT (2001) A natural history of cleidocranial dysplasia. Am J Med Genet 104:1–6

Mundlos S (1999) Cleidocranial dysplasia: clinical and molecular genetics. J Med Genet 36:177–182

Spranger JW, Brill PWE, Poznanski A (2002) Bone dysplasia, 2nd edn., Elsevier GmbH, Urban & Fischer, Munich

Stewart PA, Wallerstein R, Moran E, Lee MJ (2000) Early prenatal diagnosis of cleidocranial dysplasia. Ultrasound Obstet Gynecol 15:154–158

Unger S, Mornet E, Mundlos S, Blaser S, Cole DEC (2002) Severe cleidocranial dysplasia can mimic hypophosphatasia. Eur J Pediatr 161:623–626

Zhou G, Chen Y, Zhou L et al (1999) CBFA1 Mutation analysis and functional correlation with phenotypic variability in cleidocranial dysplasia. Hum Mol Genet 8:2311–2316

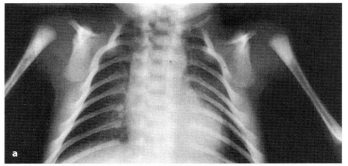

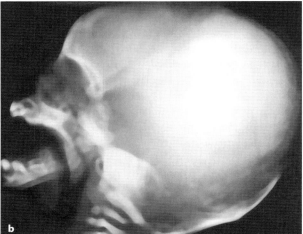

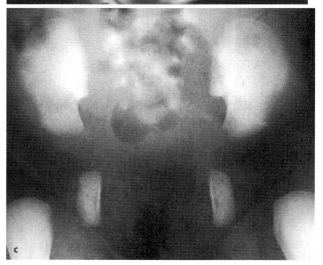

Fig. 3.51a–c. *Cleidocranial dysplasia.* Full-term newborn. **a** The clavicle is absent on the right side and hypoplastic on the left. **b** Ossification of the calvaria is deficient. Numerous wormian bones are present in the occipital and parietal bones. **c** The pubic bones are not ossified and the space between the os sacrum and iliac bones is wide. (From: Spranger et al.: Bone Dysplasias, 2nd edn., 2002, with kind permission from Elsevier GmbH, Urban & Fischer, Munich)

Mesomelic Dysplasia, Langer Type   MIM 249700

Synonyms: Mesomelic dwarfism of the hypoplastic ulna, fibula, and mandible type; homozygous dyschondrosteosis.

Major Radiographic Features:
- Disproportionate shortness of the mesial segments of the extremities
- Distal hypoplasia of the ulna; radial bowing of the radius
- Short tibia; hypoplasia of the proximal fibula

Mode of Inheritance: Autosomal recessive; parents have Madelung deformity and short stature (Dyschondrosteosis).

Molecular Basis: Deletion or mutation of the *SHOX* gene in the pseudoautosomal region of the X and Y chromosomes.

Prenatal Diagnosis: Short extremities are detected by ultrasound. Madelung deformity in both parents should alert to a 25% risk of Langer mesomelic dysplasia in the fetus.

Differential Diagnosis: *Dyschondrosteosis* is a milder condition without excessive shortness of the fibula. Numerous *other mesomelic dysplasias* are differentiated on the basis of associated features including tibio/talar fusion (Kantaputra dysplasia), short metacarpal/metatarsal bones (Ferraz dysplasia), short phalanges (Robinow syndrome, Osebold dysplasia), and others (see Spranger et al. 2002, p. 335).

Prognosis: Intellectual and motor development are normal, adult height is reduced.

Remarks: Langer mesomelic dysplasia is the homozygous form of Leri-Weill dyschondrosteosis.

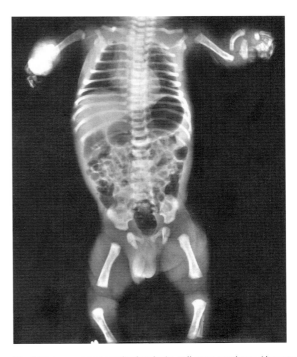

Fig. 3.52. *Langer mesomelic dysplasia.* Full-term newborn. Abnormalities of the upper extremity are best seen on the left side, which shows a short, thick ulna, and proximal hypoplasia and bowing of the radius. Absence of the proximal third of the fibula is noted. The tibiae are short

References

Langer LO (1967) Mesomelic dwarfism of the hypoplastic ulna, fibula, mandible type. Radiology 654–660

Shears DJ, Guillen-Navarro E, Sempere-Miralles M et al (2002) Pseudodominant inheritance of Langer mesomelic dysplasia caused by a SHOX homeobox missense mutation. Am J Med Genet 110 : 153–158

Spranger J, Brill PW, Polznanski AK (2002) Bone dysplasias. Urban and Fischer, Munich

Zador IE, Quareshi F, Budev H, Quigg H, Nadler HL (1988) Ultrasonographic prenatal diagnosis and fetal pathology of Langer mesomelic dwarfism. Am J Med Genet 31 : 915–920

Zinn AR, Wei F, Zhang L et al (2002) Complete SHOX deficiency causes Langer mesomelic dysplasia AM J Med Genet 110 : 158–162

Robinow Syndrome   MIM 180700, 268310

Synonym: Fetal face syndrome.

Major Radiographic Features:
- Short ulna and radius; dislocation of the radial head in severe cases
- Occasionally bifid phalanges
- Short tibia and fibula
- Frequently hemivertebrae and fusion of vertebral bodies in severe cases

Mode of Inheritance: Autosomal recessive and autosomal dominant.

Molecular Basis: Autosomal recessive Robinow syndrome is caused by homozygous loss-of-function mutations of the *ROR2* gene located on chromosome 9q22. The protein product of this gene is a cell membrane receptor involved in extracellular protein interactions and intracellular signaling pathways. The molecular defect in the autosomal dominant variety is unknown.

Prenatal Diagnosis: In a severely affected fetus sonography disclosed short extremities and increased nuchal translucency in the 12th week of gestation. Molecular analysis can be attempted in familial, autosomal recessive cases with known mutations.

Differential Diagnosis: In *Langer mesomelic dysplasia*, ulna and fibula are more severely shortened than radius and tibia. *Omodysplasia* differs by the distally tapered, short humerus and femur. *Other mesomelic dysplasias* are ruled out by the different aspect of the bones of the shanks and forearms, associated acral abnormalities, and clinical features.

Prognosis: Mortality is approximately 10% in autosomal recessive cases and not elevated in the dominant variety. Affected individuals are short and may have associated anomalies including genital hypoplasia and renal and cardiac defects. Intelligence is usually normal.

Remarks: Autosomal recessive Robinow syndrome tends to be more severe than the autosomal dominant variety with more severe mesomelic shortening, more frequent vertebral anomalies, and 10% mortality (probably due to associated defects), but there is considerable overlap between the two forms. Heterozygotes with the mutated *ROR2* gene may have short or absent middle and distal phalanges (brachydactyly B).

References

Afzal AR, Jeffery S (2003) One gene, two phenotypes: ROR2 mutations in autosomal recessive Robinow syndrome and autosomal dominant brachydactyly type B. Hum Mutat 22:1–11

Giedion AM, Battaglia GF, Bellini F, Fanconi G (1975) The radiological diagnosis of the fetal face (=Robinow) syndrome (mesomelic dwarfism and small genitalia.). Helv Paediat Acta 30:409–423

Patton MA, Afzal AR (2002) Robinow syndrome. J Med Genet 39:305–310

Percin EF, Guvenal T, Cetin A et al (2001) First trimester diagnosis of Robinow syndrome. Fetal Diagn Ther 16:308–311

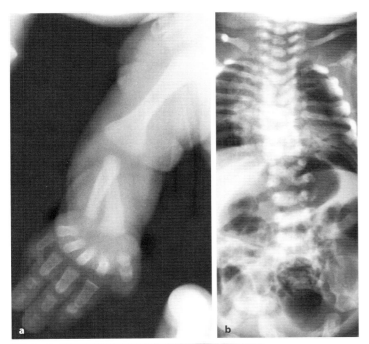

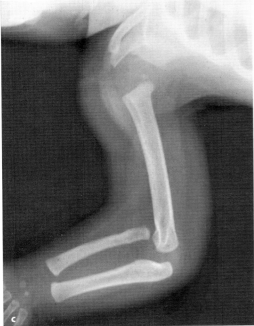

Fig. 3.53a–c. *Robinow syndrome.* **a, b** *Autosomal recessive.* Full-term newborn. There is dysspondylosis with numerous hemivertebrae and fused vertebrae. Ulna and radius are short and thick. **c** *Autosomal dominant*, 3-month. Milder shortening of ulna and radius than in **b**; dislocated head of radius

Nievergelt Syndrome   MIM 163400

Major Radiographic Features:
- Very short, triangular, or rhomboid tibiae; sometimes similar abnormality of the radii
- Less marked shortening of the fibulae and ulnae

Mode of Inheritance: Autosomal dominant.

Prenatal Diagnosis: Short mesial segments of the extremities can be detected by sonography.

Differential Diagnosis: In *Langer mesomelic dysplasia* the fibula and ulna are more severely affected than the tibia and radius. A short tibia and radius are found in *other mesomelic dysplasias* (for reference see Spranger et al. 2002, p. 335).

Prognosis: Development and life expectancy are normal.

Remarks: There is considerable intrafamilial variability of expression.

References

Burnstein MI, Desmet AA, Breed AL, Thomax JR, Hafez GR (1989) Longitudinal tibial epiphyseal bracket in Nievergelt syndrome. Skeletal Radiol 18 : 121–125

Hess OM, Goebel NH, Strewuli R (1978) Familiärer mesomeler Kleinwuchs (Nievergelt Syndrom). Schweiz Med Wochenschr 108 : 1202–1206

Monga P, Swamy MKS, Rao KS (2003) Rhomboid shaped tibia and hypoplastic fibula: a variant of Nievergelt syndrome. Am J Med Genet 118A : 394–397

Spranger JW, Brill PW, Poznanski AK (2002) Bone dysplasias. Urban and Fischer, Munich

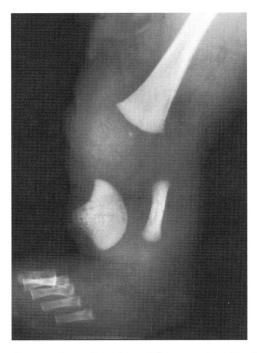

Fig. 3.54. *Nievergelt syndrome*, full-term newborn. The tibia is very short and halberd shaped. The fibula is less markedly shortened and straight

Grebe Dysplasia   MIM 200700, 201250, 228900

Synonym: Brazilian achondrogenesis, which includes Hunter-Thompson syndrome, Du Pan syndrome; CDMP1 dysplasia (Grebe, Hunter-Thompson, Du Pan types).

Major Radiographic Features:

- Variable shortness of femur and humerus
- Short ulna, bowed radius, radioulnar dislocation in severe (Grebe) and moderately severe (Hunter-Thompson) subtypes, almost normal radius and ulna in mild (Du Pan) subtype
- Short, misshapen metacarpals and metatarsals; hypoplastic, misshaped, or absent phalanges
- Short and broad tibiae
- Fibular a/hypoplasia
- Normal craniofacial and axial skeleton

Mode of Inheritance: Autosomal recessive.

Molecular Basis: Grebe dysplasia is caused by mutations of the *CDMP1* gene located on chromosome 20q11.2 coding for cartilage-derived morphogenetic protein-1, a signaling molecule involved in the patterning of the appendicular skeleton, in chondrogenesis, and in longitudinal bone growth.

Prenatal Diagnosis: Short limbs and fingers are detectable by ultrasound. Molecular analysis is possible in families with a known mutation.

Differential Diagnosis: *Langer mesomelic dysplasia, Nievergelt dysplasia,* and *other mesomelic bone dysplasias* differ by the more normal aspect of the hands and feet.

Prognosis: The patients' major handicap is short stature. Their psychomotor and intellectual development is normal.

Remarks: Allelic mutations of the *CDMP1* gene lead to a wide spectrum of disorders formerly thought to represent different entities (i.e., Grebe, Hunter-Thompson, and Du Pan dysplasia). These three disorders differ mostly by the degree of involvement of the long tubular bones. Heterozygote carriers of the *CDMP1* mutation may have brachydactyly C (short middle phalanges, misshaped extraphalangeal ossification centers).

References

Al-Yahyaee SAS, Al-Kindi MN, Habbal O, Kumar DS (2003) Clinical and molecular analysis of Grebe acromesomelic dysplasia in an Omani family. Am J Med Genet 121A: 9–14

Faiyaz-Ul-Haque M, Ahmad W, Zaidi SHE et al (2002) Mutations in the cartilage-derived morphogenetic protein-1 (CDMP1) gene in a kindred affected with fibular hypoplasia, and complex brachydactyly (Du Pan syndrome) Clin Genet 61: 454–458

Stelzer C, Winterpacht A, Spranger J, Zabel B (2003) Grebe dysplasia and the spectrum of CDMP1 mutations. Pediatr Pathol Mol Med 22: 77–85

Thomas JT, Liln K, Nandekar M et al (1996) A human chondrodysplasia due to a mutation in a TGT-beta superfamily member. Nature Genet 12: 315–317

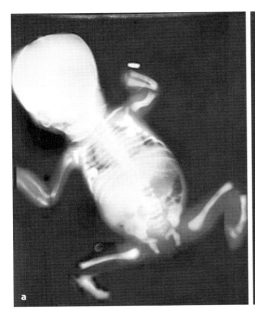
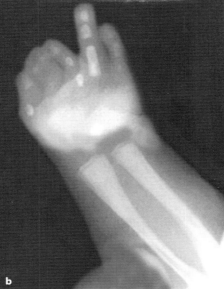

Fig. 3.55a, b. *Du Pan variety of CDMP1 dysplasia.* 38 weeks' gestation. **a** The humeri are short and bowed on the left but not on the right side. The tibiae are short and anteriorly bowed with complete absence of the fibulae. **b** The metacarpals are not ossified. Three phalanges are seen in the index finger; those in the other fingers are small, misshaped, or not ossified. There is an extra bone in the carpal region

Infantile Osteopetrosis   MIM 259700, 259720

Synonym: Infantile malignant osteopetrosis, including lethal osteopetrosis.

Major Radiographic Features:
- Generalized increased bone density
- Metaphyseal undermodeling
- Radiolucent bands at the long bone metaphyses

Mode of Inheritance: Autosomal recessive; nonallelic heterogeneity.

Molecular Basis:
A *TCIRG1* (T-cell-immune regulator 1) gene located on chromosome 11q13.4–13.5
B *CLC7* (Chloride channel 7) gene located on chromosome 16p13

Prenatal Diagnosis: If the mutation is known from previous siblings, molecular diagnosis is possible.

Differential Diagnosis: The bone changes in *Raine syndrome* are almost indistinguishable from those in infantile osteopetrosis. The lethal autosomal recessive disorder differs by the craniofacial appearance with bulging fontanelles, proptosis, hypoplastic nose, and micrognathia. In contrast to infantile osteopetrosis, the outer contours of the long bones are irregular due to excessive subperiosteal bone formation. *Other forms of osteopetrosis* including autosomal dominant and autosomal recessive late types, *carboanhydrase deficiency, pyknodysostosis, osteomesopyknosis.* or *dysosteosclerosis* may manifest in the neonate with comparatively mild sclerosis. They are rarely recognized in fetal life or the neonatal period.

Prognosis: Neonatal mortality is increased. Surviving infants may reach adulthood after bone marrow transplantation in early childhood.

Remarks: The combination of infantile osteopetrosis with absence of the corpus callosum and neuraxonal dystrophy was reported by Rees et al. in 1995. This may be a separate entity or a contiguous gene syndrome combining manifestations of infantile osteopetrosis and neuraxonal dystrophy.

References

Chalhoub N, Benachenhou N, Rajapurohitam V (2003) Grey-lethal mutation induces severe malignant autosomal recessive osteopetrosis in mouse and human. Nature Med 9:399–406

Loria-Cortes R, Quesada-Calvo E, Cordero-Chaverri E (1977) Osteopetrosis in children. A report on 26 cases. J Pediatr 91:43–47

Ogur G, Ogur E, Celasun B et al (1995) Prenatal diagnosis of autosomal recessive osteopetrosis, infantile type, by x-ray evaluation. Prenatal Diag 15:477–481

Rees et al (1995) Pediatr Neurosurg 22:321

Sobacchi C, Frattini A, Orchard P et al (2003) The mutational spectrum of human malignant autosomal recessive osteopetrosis. Hum Mol Genet 15:1767–1773

Wilson CJ, Vellodid A (2000) Autosomal recessive osteopetrosis: diagnosis, management and outcome. Arch Dis Child 83:449–452

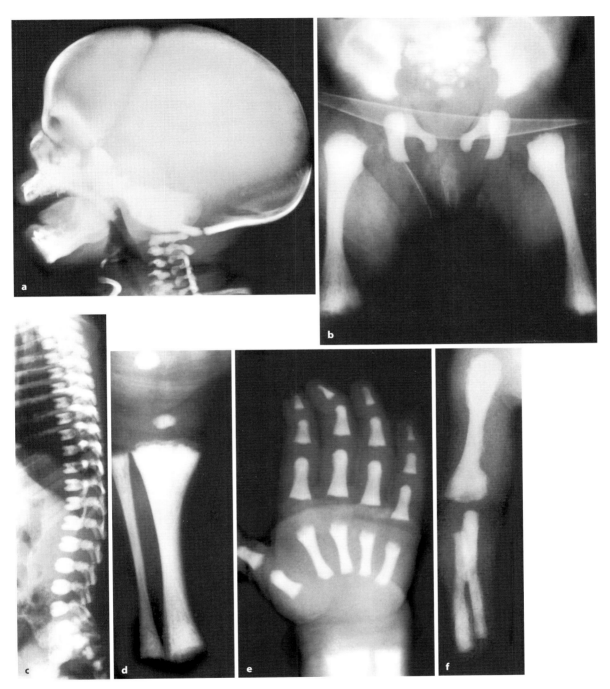

Fig. 3.56a–f. *Infantile osteopetrosis*, full-term newborn. **a** The base of the skull, facial bones, and part of the calvaria are sclerotic. **b** The vertebrae are normally formed and dense. **c, d** Pelvis and long tubular bones are homogeneously sclerotic with absent corticomedullary demarcation and lack of normal metaphyseal modeling. Note slightly irregular appearance of the proximal tibial metaphysis, which later may develop into "osteopetrorickets". **e** The short tubular bones are normally shaped and dense. **f** *Raine syndrome.* Bone density is increased as in infantile osteopetrosis, but, in addition, the contours of the long bones are irregular due to excessive subperiosteal bone formation. (Courtesy of Dr. K. Kozlowski, Sidney)

Blomstrand Syndrome   MIM168468

Major Radiographic Features:
- Generalized sclerosis
- Small facial bone
- Short and broad ribs
- Tubular bones with mushroomed ends and very short, sometimes bowed or kinked diaphyses
- Advanced bone maturation

Mode of Inheritance: Autosomal recessive.

Molecular Basis: Mutations of the *PTHR1* gene located on chromosome 3p22-p21.1 encoding a receptor for both parathyroid hormone and parathyroid hormone-related protein, resulting in the inactivation of the PTH receptor.

Prenatal Diagnosis: Fetal sonography showed polyhydramnios and very short limbs at 19 weeks' gestation. In familial cases, molecular diagnosis should be possible.

Differential Diagnosis: In *infantile osteosclerosis* the tubular bones are straight with less severe metaphyseal widening.

Prognosis: All known patients were stillborn or died shortly after birth.

Remarks: Pathogenetically, Jansen and Blomstrand dysplasia are mirror images. Lack of function of the parathyroid hormone receptor causes Blomstrand dysplasia, its constitutive activation Jansen metaphyseal dysplasia.

References
Blomstrand S, Classon I, Säve-Söderbergh J (1985) A case of lethal congenital dwarfism with accelerated skeletal maturation. Pediatr Radiol 15:141–143

Jobert AS, Zhang P, Couvineau A et al (1998) Absence of functional receptors for parathyroid hormone and parathyro8d hormone-related peptide in Blomstrand chondrodysplasia. J Clin Invest 102:34–40

Loshkajian A, Roume J, Stanescu V et al (1997) Familial Blomstrand chondrodysplasia with advanced skeletal maturation. Am J Med Genet 71:283–288

Oostra RJ, van der Haren HJ, Rijnders WPHA et al (3000) Blomstrand osteochondrodysplasia: three novel cases and histological evidence for heterogeneity. Virchows Arch 436:28–35

Spranger JW, Brill PWE, Poznanski A (2002) Bone dysplasia, 2nd edn., Elsevier GmbH, Urban & Fischer, Munich

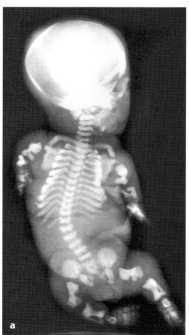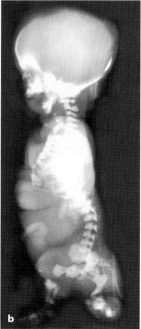

Fig. 3.57a, b. *Blomstrand dysplasia*, 32 weeks' gestation. The skeleton is sclerotic. The viscerocranium is disproportionately small. The chest is small with thick clavicles and ribs. The tubular bones are very short with bowed or kinked diaphyses and wide ends. Advanced bone maturation is best appreciated in the tarsus. (From: Spranger et al.: Bone Dysplasias, 2nd edn., 2002, with kind permission from Elsevier GmbH, Urban & Fischer, Munich)

Lenz-Majewski Hyperostotic Dysplasia   MIM 151050

Synonym: Lenz-Majewski syndrome; Lenz-Majewski hyperostotic dwarfism.

Major Radiographic Features:

- Hyperdensity of the cranial base and facial bones
- Mild hyperostosis of the clavicles and ribs
- Mild hyperostosis of the tubular bones
- Irregular shortening of the metacarpals, defective ossification and fusion of the proximal and middle phalanges especially on the ulnar side

Mode of Inheritance: Uncertain, possibly autosomal dominant.

Molecular Basis: Unknown.

Prenatal Diagnosis: Uncertain.

Differential Diagnosis: The *physiologic skeletal hyperdensity* of the premature infant is less severe and disappears during the first weeks of life. More severe sclerosis and tubular undermodeling are found *in infantile osteopetrosis* and *Blomstrand dysplasia*. The aberrant metacarpal and phalangeal ossification in the Lenz-Majewski syndrome assists in its differentiation from the former and from disorders with mildly increased bone density such as *pyknodysostosis, osteopetrosis with renal tubular acidosis* (carboanhydrase deficiency), or *dysosteosclerosis*.

Prognosis: Neonatal mortality is increased. Survivors have been followed up to adulthood with mental retardation and short stature.

References

Gorlin RJ, Whitley CM (1983) Lenz-Majewski syndrome. Radiology 149:129–131

Robinow M, Johanson AJ, Smith TH (1977) The Lenz-Majewski hyperostotic dwarfism: a syndrome of multiple congenital anomalies, mental retardation, and progressive skeletal sclerosis. J Pediatr 91:417–421

Saraiva JM (2000) Dysgenesis of corpus callosum in Lenz-Majewski hyperostotic dwarfism. Am J Med Genet 91:198–200

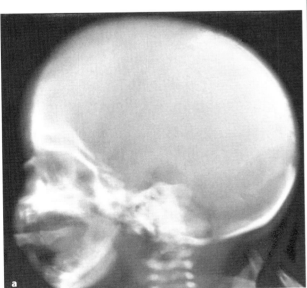
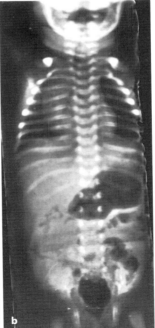

Fig. 3.58a–d. *Lenz-Majewski Syndrome.* Full-term newborn. **a** There is mild hyperdensity of the cranial base, facial bones, and part of the cranial vault. **b** The bone density is increased in the clavicles, ribs, and pedicles

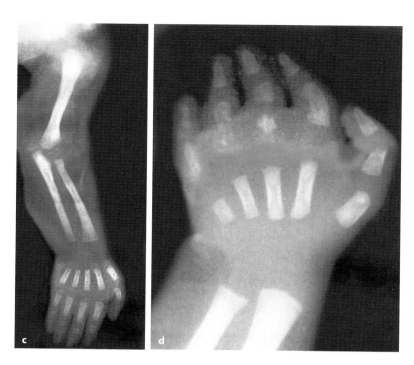

Fig. 3.58. c Patchy hyperdensities are present in the long tubular bones. **d** The first and fifth metacarpals are short. There is erratic ossification and partial fusion of the proximal and middle phalanges of the 2nd to 5th fingers. Fusion of the proximal and middle phalanx of the index finger is complete

Appendix

Amelia – Amputation – Phocomelia

Diagnosis	Skull	Spine	Humerus
Acrofacial dysostosis, type Rodriguez			×
Amelia, autosomal recessive			×
Amnion disruption sequence; ADAM; Limb-body wall complex	×	×	
Diabetic embryopathy		×	
DK phocomelia; Phocomelia-encephalocele-thrombocytopenia-urogenital malformation; von Voss-Cherstvoy syndrome	×		×
Oromandibula-limb hypogenesis syndromes incl. Hanhart syndrome			
Roberts (pseudothalidomide) syndrome	×		×
Schinzel-Giedion syndrome	×		
Sirenomelia		×	
Splenogonadal fusion – limb defects	×	×	
Tetraamelia with multiple malformations	×	×	
Thalidomide embryopathy			×
Thrombocytopenia-absent radius (TAR) syndrome (severe form)			×

Radius: Aplasia, Hypoplasia ± Aplasia of Thumb [1]

Diagnosis	Skull	Spine	Humerus
Acrofacial dysostosis, type Rodriguez			×
Amnion disruption sequence; ADAM; Limb, body wall complex	×	×	
Baller-Gerold syndrome	×		
Brachmann-de Lange syndrome			
Chromosome abnormality; Trisomy 18 (Edward syndrome)	×	×	
Chromosome 13 q syndrome			
Fanconi pancytopenia; TAR			
Fetal valproate syndrome	×		
Fryns syndrome – acral defects			
Goldenhar syndrome	×	×	
Holt-Oram (cardiomelic) syndrome			×
Mesomelic dysplasias			
MURCS association		×	
Nager acrofacial dysostosis	×		
Poland syndrome		×	
Roberts (pseudothalidomide) syndrome	×		×
Sirenomelia		×	
VACTERL association		×	

Radius	Ulna	Femur	Tibia	Fibula	Hands/Feet	Others
×	×			×	×	Hypoplastic scapulae
×	×	×	×	×	×	
		×			×	
		×	×		×	Cardiac defects, anal atresia
×	×				×	Genitourinary and cardiac anomalies
					×	Microglossia, transverse limb reduction
×	×	×	×	×	×	Cystic hygroma
×	×		×	×		Bowing of long bones
×		×	×	×	×	Anal atresia
					×	Micrognathia, transverse limb reduction
						Nearly totally absent limbs
×	×	×	×	×		Defects mostly proximal
×	×				×	Present thumb

Radius	Ulna	Femur	Tibia	Fibula	Hands/Feet	Others
×	×			×	×	Hypoplastic scapulae
×					×	Ventral wall defect
×					×	
×	×				×	
×			×		×	
					×	Growth retardation
×					×	TAR: present thumbs
×					×	
×					×	Diaphragmatic hernia
×						
×	×				×	Heart lesions (ASD, VSD)
×	×		×	×	×	See p. 155
×					×	
×	×					
		×			×	Aplasia of pectoralis muscle
×	×	×	×	×	×	Cystic hygroma
×		×	×	×	×	Anal atresia
×			×	×	×	Intestinal atresias

Radio-ulnar Synostosis

Diagnosis	Skull	Spine	Humerus
Cenani-Lenz syndrome		×	
Cloverleaf skull – limb anomaly, type Holtermüller-Wiedemann	×		
Chromosome abnormality; Trisomy 18 (Edward syndrome)	×	×	
Chromosome abnormality; Klinefelter syndrome			
Fetal alcohol syndrome		(×)	
Holt-Oram (cardiomelic) syndrome			×
Nager acrofacial dysostosis	×		
Radio-ulnar synostosis, autosomal dominant			

Ulna: Aplasia, Hypoplasia

Diagnosis	Skull	Spine	Humerus
Acrofacial dysostosis with post-axial defects	×		
Acrofacial dysostosis, type Rodriguez			×
Brachmann-de Lange syndrome			
Femur-fibula-ulna complex			×
Fetal alcohol syndrome		(×)	
Grebe syndrome			×
Holt-Oram (cardiomelic) syndrome			×
Leri-Weill dyschondrosteosis			
Mesomelic dysplasias			
Neu-Laxova syndrome	×		
Neurofibromatosis 1			
Roberts (pseudothalidomide) syndrome	×		×
Thrombocytopenia-absent radius (TAR) syndrome			
Ulnar-mammary syndrome type Pallister			
Weyers syndrome			

Radius	Ulna	Femur	Tibia	Fibula	Hands/Feet	Others
×	×				×	
×	×					
×	×		×		×	
×	×					
×	×				×	Growth retardation
×	×				×	Heart lesions (ASD, VSD)
×	×					
×	×					

Radius	Ulna	Femur	Tibia	Fibula	Hands/Feet	Others
	×				×	
×	×			×	×	Hypoplastic scapula
×	×				×	
	×	×		×		Synostosis around the elbow
	×				×	Growth retardation
×	×	×	×	×	×	See p. 159
×	×				×	Heart lesions (ASD, VSD)
×	×			×		
×	×		×	×	×	See p. 155 ff
×	×				×	
×	×	×	×			Pseudarthrosis
×	×	×	×	×	×	Cystic hygroma
×	×					Present thumb
	×				×	Anal atresia
	×			×	×	

Humerus: Aplasia, Hypoplasia

Diagnosis	Skull	Spine	Humerus
Acrofacial dysostosis, type Rodriguez			×
Atelosteogenesis and related OCDs		×	×
Brachmann-de Lange syndrome			
CHILD syndrome			×
Chondrodysplasia punctata, rhizomelic type		×	×
Chondrodysplasia punctata, tibia-metacarpal type			×
DK phocomelia; Phocomelia-encephalocele-thrombocytopenia-urogenital malformation; von Voss-Cherstvoy syndrome	×		×
Femur-fibula-ulna complex			×
Fetal thalidomide			×
Fetal valproate syndrome	×		×
Holt-Oram (cardiomelic) syndrome			×
Omodysplasia			×
Oromandibula-limb hypogenesis syndromes incl. Hanhart syndrome			×
Thrombocytopenia-absent radius (TAR) syndrome (severe form)			×

Tibia: Aplasia, Hypoplasia

Diagnosis	Skull	Spine	Humerus
Amnion disruption sequence; ADAM; Limb, body wall complex	×	×	
Chondrodysplasia punctata, tibia-metacarpal type			
Chromosome abnormality; Trisomy 18 (Edward syndrome)	×	×	
Grebe syndrome			×
Mesomelic dysplasias			
Mesomelic dwarfism of hypoplastic tibia-radius type			
Neurofibromatosis 1			
Split hands/feet, tibial defect			
Tibial hemimelia			
Tibial hypoplasia, polydactyly and triphalangeal thumb (Werner)			
VACTERL association		×	

Radius	Ulna	Femur	Tibia	Fibula	Hands/Feet	Others
×	×			×	×	Hypoplastic scapulae
×	×	×		×	×	See p. 148
×	×				×	
×	×	×	×	×		Unilateral
		×				See p. 142
		×	×		×	
×	×				×	Genitourinary and cardiac anomalies
	×	×		×		Synostosis around the elbow
×	×	×	×	×		Defects mostly proximal
×					×	
×	×				×	Heart lesions (ASD, VSD)
×	×	×	×	×		See p. 152
					×	Microglossia, transverse limb reduction
×	×				×	Present thumb

Radius	Ulna	Femur	Tibia	Fibula	Hands/Feet	Others
			×		×	Ventral wall defect, transverse reductions
		×	×		×	
×			×		×	
×	×	×	×	×	×	See p. 159
×	×		×	×	×	See p. 155
×			×			
×	×	×	×			Pseudarthrosis
	×	×	×		×	
			×		×	
×	×		×		×	Mesomelic dysplasia
×			×	×	×	Intestinal atresias

Fibula: Aplasia, Hypoplasia

Diagnosis	Skull	Spine	Humerus
Acrofacial dysostosis, type Rodriguez			×
Camptomelic dysplasia		×	×
Chondroectodermal dysplasia; Ellis van-Creveld			
De la Chapelle dysplasia		×	×
Du Pan brachydactyly, fibular aplasia			
Ectrodactyly-fibular aplasia			
Femur-fibula-ulna complex			×
Femoral hypoplasia, unusual facies syndrome	×		
Fibular aplasia/hypoplasia			
Limb/pelvis hypoplasia/aplasia syndrome		×	
Mesomelic dysplasias			
Seckel syndrome	×		
VACTERL-Association		×	

Femur: Aplasia, Hypoplasia

Diagnosis	Skull	Spine	Humerus
Diabetic embryopathy		×	
Ectrodactyly-tibial hypoplasia			
Femoral hypoplasia, unusual facies syndrome	×		
Femur-fibula-ulna complex			×
Limb, body wall complex		×	
Limb/pelvis hypoplasia/aplasia syndrome		×	
Omodysplasia			×
Proximal focal femoral deficiency			

Radius	Ulna	Femur	Tibia	Fibula	Hands/Feet	Others
×	×			×	×	Hypoplastic scapula
×	×	×	×	×	×	Pear-shaped ilia; see p. 114
		×	×	×	×	See p. 137
		×	×	×	×	See p. 137
				×	×	Dislocation of great joint; see p. 159
	×			×	×	
	×	×		×		Synostosis around the elbow
		×	×	×	×	Micrognathia
				×		
×	×	×	×	×	×	Hypoplastic pelvis
×	×		×	×	×	See p. 155 ff
				×		Severe growth retardation
×			×	×	×	Intestinal atresias

Radius	Ulna	Femur	Tibia	Fibula	Hands/Feet	Others
		×	×		×	Cardiac defects, anal atresia
		×	×		×	
		×	×	×	×	Micrognathia
	×	×		×		Synostosis around the elbow
×		×			×	Bladder exstrophy
×	×	×	×	×	×	Hypoplastic pelvis
×	×	×	×	×		See p. 152
		×				

Stippled Epiphyses – Stippled Ossification of Cartilage
(for skeletal dyslasias with punctate calcifications see p. 162 ff)

Diagnosis	Skull	Spine	Humerus
Chromosome abnormality Triploidy		×	
Chromosome abnormality; Trisomy 13	×	×	
Chromosome abnormality; Trisomy 18 (Edward syndrome)	×	×	
Chromosome abnormality; Trisomy 21		×	
Chromosome abnormality; Turner syndrome			
Fetal alcohol syndrome		(×)	
Hydantoin embryopathy	×		
Smith-Lemli-Opitz syndrome	×		
Warfarin embryopathy	×		
Zellweger syndrome	×		

Absent Hands/Feet

Diagnosis	Skull	Spine	Humerus
Acheiropodia			
Amnion disruption sequence; ADAM; Limb, body wall complex	×	×	
Brachmann-de Lange syndrome			
Femur-fibula-ulna complex			×
Holoprosencephaly-transverse limb defect			
Oromandibula-limb hypogenesis syndromes incl. Hanhart syndrome			

Radius	Ulna	Femur	Tibia	Fibula	Hands/Feet	Others
						Severe growth retardation
					×	Omphalocele
×			×		×	
					×	
					×	Hygroma
	×				×	Growth retardation
					×	Stippled epiphyses
					×	Growth retardation
					×	Stippled calcifications
						Stippled calcifications around the pelvis

Radius	Ulna	Femur	Tibia	Fibula	Hands/Feet	Others
×	×		×	×	×	
		×			×	
×	×				×	
	×	×		×	×	Synostosis around the elbow
					×	
					×	Microglossia, transverse limb reduction

Split/Cleft/Ectrodactyly of Hands and/or Feet

Diagnosis	Skull	Spine	Humerus
Acro-renal-mandibular syndrome	×	×	
Brachmann-de Lange syndrome			
Chromosome abnormality; Trisomy 13	×	×	
Chromosome abnormality; Trisomy 18 (Edward syndrome)	×	×	
DK phocomelia; Phocomelia-encephalocele-thrombocytopenia-urogenital malformation; von Voss-Cherstvoy syndrome	×		×
Ectrodactyly-Ectodermal dysplasia-Clefting syndrome	×		
Ectrodactyly-fibular aplasia			
Ectrodactyly, isolated			
Ectrodactyly-tibial hypoplasia			
Femur-fibula-ulna complex			×
Holoprosencephaly-hypertelorism-ectrodactyly syndrome	×		
Monodactylous ectrodactyly and bifid femur; Wolfgang-Gollop syndrome		×	
Oromandibula-limb hypogenesis syndromes incl. Hanhart syndrome			

Preaxial Polydactyly of Hands and/or Feet

Diagnosis	Skull	Spine	Humerus
Aase syndrome; Diamond-Blackfan syndrome; Anemia and triphalangeal thumbs			
Acrocallosal syndrome	×		
Carpenter syndrome; Acrocephalopolysyndactyly, type 2; Chromosome abnormalities	×		
Diabetic embryopathy		×	
Greig cephalopolysyndactyly	×		
Holt-Oram (cardiomelic) syndrome			×
Hydrolethalus syndrome	×		
Orofacial digital syndromes	×		
Pfeiffer syndrome; Acrocephalosyndactyly V	×		
Pseudo-trisomy 13 syndrome	×	×	
Short rib-polydactyly, different types		×	×
Townes-Brocks syndrome			

Radius	Ulna	Femur	Tibia	Fibula	Hands/Feet	Others
×			×		×	Severe hypoplasia of mandible
×	×				×	
					×	Omphalocele
×			×		×	
×	×				×	Genitourinary and cardiac anomalies
					×	Cleft lip/palate, renal dysplasia
	×			×	×	
					×	
		×	×		×	
	×	×		×		Synostosis around the elbow
×	×				×	Cleft lip,
×	×	×	×	×	×	
					×	Microglossia, transverse limb reduction
					×	
					×	Macrosomy at birth
					×	
		×	×		×	Cardiac defects, anal atresia
					×	
×	×				×	Heart lesions (ASD, VSD)
					×	Micrognathia
			×		×	
					×	
×	×				×	Omphalocele
×	×	×	×	×	×	See p. 133 ff; Very short ribs
					×	Anal atresia

Postaxial Polydactyly of Hands and/or Feet

Diagnosis	Skull	Spine	Humerus
Acrocallosal syndrome	×		
Asphyxiating thoracic dystrophy, Jeune syndrome			
Acrocephalopolydactyly II (Carpenter)	×		
Chromosome abnormality; Trisomy 13	×	×	
Elejalde syndrome	×		×
Ellis van-Creveld syndrome Chondroectodermal dysplasia			
Focal dermal hypoplasia; Goltz syndrome			
Grebe syndrome			×
Greig cephalopolysyndactyly	×		
Hydrolethalus syndrome	×		
Isolated defect			
Meckel-Gruber syndrome	×		
Orofacial digital syndromes	×		
Pallister-Hall syndrome			
Pseudo-trisomy 13 syndrome	×	×	
Short rib-polydactyly syndrome, different types		×	×
Simpson-Golabi-Behmel syndrome	×	×	
Smith-Lemli-Opitz syndrome	×		

Premature Cranial Synostosis/Cloverleaf Skull

Diagnosis	Skull	Spine	Humerus
Acrocephalosyndactyly I (Apert)			
Acrocephalosyndactyly V (Pfeiffer)			
Acrocephalopolydactyly II (Carpenter)	×		
Amnion disruption sequence; ADAM; Limb, body wall complex	×	×	
Antley-Bixler syndrome	×		×
Baller-Gerold syndrome	×		
Cloverleaf skull – limb anomaly, type Holtermüller-Wiedemann	×		
M. Crouzon	×		
Osteocraniostenosis	×		×
Osteoglophonic dysplasia	×	×	×
Seckel syndrome	×		
Short rib-polydactyly, Beemer-Langer type	×	×	×
Thanatophoric dysplasia II	×		

Radius	Ulna	Femur	Tibia	Fibula	Hands/Feet	Others
					×	Macrosomy at birth
					×	See p. 135; Narrow thorax
					×	
					×	Omphalocele
×	×	×	×	×	×	Cystic hygroma
		×	×		×	See p. 137
					×	Clavicular hypoplasia
×	×	×	×	×	×	See p. 159
					×	
					×	Micrognathia
					×	
					×	Growth retardation
			×		×	
					×	Anal atresia
×	×				×	Omphalocele
×	×	×	×	×	×	See p. 133 ff; Very short ribs
					×	Hydrops fetalis
					×	Growth retardation

Radius	Ulna	Femur	Tibia	Fibula	Hands/Feet	Others
					×	
		×			×	
×						See p. 116; Fractures
×					×	
×	×					
×	×	×	×	×		See p. 127; Fractures
		×			×	
				×		Severe growth retardation
×	×	×	×	×	×	See p. 134; Very short ribs
						See p. 94

Un-/Hypo-ossified Calvaria (for skeletal dysplasia see p. 138, 148)

Diagnosis	Skull	Spine	Humerus
Acalvaria	×		
Aminopterin/methotrexate fetopathy	×		
Angiotensin inverting enzyme (ACE) inhibitor fetopathy	×		
Chromosome abnormality; Trisomy 13	×	×	
Chromosome abnormality; Trisomy 18 (Edward syndrome)	×	×	
Hyperparathyroidism, neonatal familial seal fractures	×		×
Hypophosphatasia, infantile form	×	×	×
Osteocraniostenosis	×		×
Osteogenesis imperfecta II	×		×

Differential Diagnosis of Encephalocele

Diagnosis	Skull	Spine	Humerus
Amnion disruption sequence; ADAM; Limb, body wall complex	×	×	
DK phocomelia; Phocomelia-encephalocele-thrombocytopenia-urogenital malformation; von Voss-Cherstvoy syndrome	×		×
Dyssegmental dysplasia; Silverman-Handmaker type; Rolland-Desbuquois type	×	×	
Incidental finding	×	×	
Iniencephaly	×	×	×
Meckel-Gruber syndrome	×		
Roberts (pseudothalidomide) syndrome	×		×
VATER association with hydrocephalus	×	×	
Walker-Warburg syndrome	×		
Warfarin embryopathy	×		

Radius	Ulna	Femur	Tibia	Fibula	Hands/Feet	Others
						Spina bifida, omphalocele
×	×					Growth retardation
						Growth retardation
					×	Omphalocele
×			×		×	
×	×	×	×	×		Subperiosteal bone resorption, metaphy-
×	×	×	×	×	×	
×	×	×	×	×		See p. 127; Fractures
×	×	×	×	×		See p. 118; Multiple fractures incl. ribs

Radius	Ulna	Femur	Tibia	Fibula	Hands/Feet	Others
		×			×	
×	×				×	Genitourinary and cardiac anomalies
×	×	×	×	×		See p. 110
						No other radiologic findings
						Omphalocele
					×	Growth retardation
×	×	×	×	×	×	Cystic hygroma
×			×	×	×	Intestinal atresias
					×	Stippled calcifications

Anencephaly/Myelomeningocele/Spina Bifida

Diagnosis	Skull	Spine	Humerus
Amnion disruption sequence; ADAM			
Limb, body wall complex	×	×	
CHILD syndrome			×
Chromosome abnormality; Trisomy 18 (Edward syndrome)	×	×	
Diabetic embryopathy		×	
Fetal aminopterin syndrome; Folate antagonist chemotherapeutic agents	×		
Fetal valproate syndrome	×		
Isolated defect with or without rachischisis	×	×	
Laterality sequence		×	
Meckel-Gruber syndrome	×		
Omphalocele-exstrophy of the bladder-imperforate anus-spinal defect (OEIS) complex;		×	
Pentalogy of Cantrell; Thoracoabdominal syndrome			
Short-rib polydactyly syndrome, type II		×	×

adius	Ulna	Femur	Tibia	Fibula	Hands/Feet	Others
		×			×	
×	×	×	×	×		Unilateral
×			×		×	
		×	×		×	Cardiac defects, anal atresia
					×	
×					×	
						Visceral heterotaxy
					×	Growth retardation
					×	Anal atresia, wide pubic distance; sternal defect, ventral wall defect
×	×	×	×	×	×	See p. 136

Vertebral Segmentation Defects/Hemivertebrae/Vertebral Fusion

Diagnosis	Skull	Spine	Humerus
Acro-renal-mandibular syndrome	×	×	
Butterfly vertebrae, isolated		×	
Camptomelic dysplasia		×	×
Chromosome abnormality; Trisomy 13	×	×	
Chromosome abnormality; Chromosome 13 q- syndrome		×	
Chromosome abnormality; Trisomy 18 (Edward syndrome)	×	×	
Chromosome abnormality; Triploidy		×	
Diabetic embryopathy		×	
Dyssegmental dysplasia; Silverman-Handmaker type; Rolland-Desbuquois type		×	
Fetal alcohol syndrome		×	
Klippel-Feil syndrome		×	
Limb/pelvis hypoplasia/aplasia syndrome; Al-Awadi/Raas-Rothschild syndrome; Schinzel phocomelia		×	
Jarcho-Levin syndrome; Spondylocostal dysostosis; Spondylothoracic dysostosis		×	
Lethal multiple pterygium syndrome; X-linked lethal multiple pterygium syndrome		×	
MURCS association		×	
Omphalocele-exstrophy of the bladder-imperforate anus-spinal defect (OEIS) complex		×	
Spinal dysraphism	×	×	
Urorectal septum malformation sequence		×	
VACTERL association		×	
VATER association with hydrocephalus	×	×	

Radius	Ulna	Femur	Tibia	Fibula	Hands/Feet	Others
×			×		×	Severe hypoplasia of mandible
×	×	×	×		×	See p. 114; Pear-shaped ilia
					×	Omphalocele
					×	Growth retardation
×			×		×	
						Severe growth retardation
		×	×		×	Cardiac defects, anal atresia
×	×	×	×	×		See p. 110
	×				×	Growth retardation
						Cervico-thoracic vertebral fusion
×	×	×	×	×	×	Hypoplastic pelvis
						Rib synostosis, defective
					×	Cystic hygroma
×					×	
					×	Anal atresia, wide pubic distance
						Hydrocephalus
×					×	Prune belly, narrow symphysis
×			×	×	×	Intestinal atresias
×			×	×	×	Intestinal atresias

Pelvic-sacral Abnormalities

Diagnosis	Skull	Spine	Humerus
Achondrogenesis, type II; Hypochondrogenesis; Lethal type II collagenopathies	×	×	×
Boomerang dysplasia	×	×	×
Camptomelic dysplasia		×	×
Cleidocranial dysostosis	×		
Currarino triad		×	
Diabetic embryopathy		×	
Axial mesodermal dysplasia spectrum	×	×	
Isolated defect		×	
Limb, body wall complex	×	×	
Limb/pelvis hypoplasia/aplasia syndrome; Al-Awadi/Raas-Rothschild syndrome		×	
Omphalocele-exstrophy of the bladder-imperforate anus-spinal defect (OEIS) complex		×	
Opsismodysplasia		×	
Schinzel-Giedion syndrome	×		
Sirenomelia		×	
Spondyloepiphyseal dysplasia congenita (SEDc)			
Spondylometepiphyseal dysplasia (Strudwick)			
Urorectal septum malformation sequence		×	
VACTERL association		×	

Coronal Clefts of Vertebral Bodies

Diagnosis	Skull	Spine	Humerus
Atelosteogenesis and related OCDs		×	×
Chondrodysplasia punctata, rhizomelic type		×	×
Chondrodysplasia punctata, tibia-metacarpal type		×	
Chromosome abnormality; Trisomy 13	×	×	
Chromosome abnormality; Trisomy 18 (Edward syndrome)	×	×	
Chromosome abnormality Trisomy 21		×	
Chromosome abnormality			
Triploidy		×	
Desbuquois syndrome		×	×
Fibrochondrogenesis		×	×
Lethal Kniest-like dysplasia	×	×	×
Short rib-polydactyly syndrome; Type I (Saldino-Noonan)		×	×

Radius	Ulna	Femur	Tibia	Fibula	Hands/Feet	Others
×	×	×	×	×	×	See p. 106
×	×	×	×	×	×	See p. 148
×	×	×	×		×	See p. 114; Pear-shaped ilia
						Clavicles and pubic bones unossified
						Asymmetric sacral defect
		×	×		×	Cardiac defects, anal atresia
					×	
		×	×	×		
		×			×	
×	×	×	×	×	×	Hypoplastic pelvis
					×	Anal atresia, wide pubic distance
					×	Retarded skeletal maturation
×	×		×	×		Bowing of long bones
×		×	×	×	×	Anal atresia
						See p. 108; unossified pubic bone
						Like SEDc
×					×	Prune belly, narrow symphysis
×			×	×	×	Intestinal atresias

Radius	Ulna	Femur	Tibia	Fibula	Hands/Feet	Others
×	×	×		×	×	See p. 148
		×				See p. 142
		×	×		×	
					×	Omphalocele
×			×		×	
					×	
						Severe growth retardation
×	×	×	×	×	×	See p. 146; Dislocations
×	×	×	×	×		See p. 101
×	×	×	×	×		See p. 108; Very wide metaphyses
×	×	×	×	×	×	See p. 133; Very short ribs

Ectopia Cordis

Diagnosis	Skull	Spine	Humerus
Amnion disruption sequence; ADAM; Limb body wall complex; Pentalogy of Cantrell; Thoracoabdominal syndrome	×	×	
Sternal malformation-vascular dysplasia association; Sternal clefts-telangiectasia/hemangiomas; Hemangiomas, cavernous of face and supraumbilical midline raphe	×		

Ventral Wall Defects/Omphalocele/Gastroschisis

Diagnosis	Skull	Spine	Humerus
Amnion disruption sequence; ADAM; Limb body wall complex	×	×	
Boomerang dysplasia	×	×	×
Chromosome abnormality; Trisomy 13	×	×	
Chromosome abnormality; Trisomy 18 (Edward syndrome)	×	×	
Elejalde syndrome	×		×
Melnick-Needles Osteodysplasty; Oto-palato-digital syndrome, type II	×	×	
Omphalocele-Exstrophy of the bladder-Imperforate anus-Spinal defect (OEIS) complex		×	
Pseudo-trisomy 13 syndrome	×	×	
Short rib-polydactyly, Beemer-Langer type		×	×
Thoracoabdominal syndrome; Pentalogy of Cantrell			

Radius	Ulna	Femur	Tibia	Fibula	Hands/Feet	Others
		×			×	Sternal defect, ventral wall defect
						Hypoplastic clavicles

Radius	Ulna	Femur	Tibia	Fibula	Hands/Feet	Others
		×			×	
×	×	×	×	×	×	See p. 148
					×	Omphalocele
×			×		×	
×	×	×	×	×		Cystic hygroma
					×	See p. 124; Thin, wavy ribs; wavy contour of long bones
					×	Anal atresia, wide pubic distance
×	×				×	Omphalocele
×	×	×	×	×	×	See p. 134; Very short ribs
						Sternal defect, ventral wall defect

Subject Index

Bold faced page numbers refer to chapters